DR WILLIAM DAVIS

WHEAT BELLY

30-MINUTE
(OR LESS!)
COOKBOOK

200 QUICK AND SIMPLE WHEAT-FREE AND GRAIN-FREE RECIPES

Thorsons
An imprint of HarperCollins*Publishers*
1 London Bridge Street
London SE1 9GF

www.harpercollins.co.uk

First published in this edition by Rodale Inc. 2013
Published in Great Britain by Thorsons 2015

1 3 5 7 9 10 8 6 4 2

Photographs © 2013 by Rodale Inc.
Photographs by Linda Pugliese
Food styling by Carrie Ann Purcell
Prop styling by Molly FitzSimons

Book design by Carol Angstadt and Amy King

A catalogue record of this book is
available from the British Library

ISBN 978-0-00-811758-0

Printed and bound in Great Britain by
Martins the Printers Ltd, Berwick-upon-Tweed

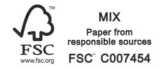

MIX
Paper from
responsible sources
FSC™ C007454

Find out more about HarperCollins and the environment at
www.harpercollins.co.uk/green

Dedicated to the
followers of *Wheat Belly,*
who asked for something
quick and easy!

CONTENTS

The Wheat-Free Lifestyle in 30 Minutes (or Less!)

WHAT CAN YOU accomplish in 30 minutes or less? In today's electronically connected world, you could publish a few comments on Facebook or post a few Tweets. Or you could walk on your treadmill for a little exercise, vacuum a couple of rooms or read another chapter in a novel. You could light some candles, darken the lights, grab your spouse . . . okay, enough of that!

Or you could take action that helps you and your family make a huge leap towards better health and prepare a meal that frees all of you from the appetite-stimulating, health-impairing, visceral fat-accumulating effects of modern wheat, enjoying quick and delicious meals that satisfy everyone weaned from the breast on up!

Since the original *Wheat Belly* was published in August 2011, followed by the *Wheat Belly Cookbook*, an international movement has been launched, a dietary revolution now embraced by millions of people who are eager to regain control over appetite, weight and health. We certainly cannot credit my charm, wit or good looks – it's the *power of the message* and the wonderful stories of success that pour in day after day, month after month, that have catapulted this message into the spotlight.

We've witnessed what happens to people who take the brave leap and do the *opposite* of what conventional advice tells us: weight and health are *transformed*. A long list of health conditions diminish or disappear. Most typically, people experience relief from acid reflux, bowel urgency, joint pain and mental 'fog'. Many diabetics become *non*-diabetic. People suffering for years with the pain and deformity of inflammatory and autoimmune conditions experience markedly reduced symptoms, or even outright cure. Depression lifts in many, while anxiety and paranoia disappear in others. The food obsessions of bulimia and binge eating disorder can dissipate within days. And, of course, pounds of fat, mostly from the inflammatory visceral fat of the abdomen, the infamous 'wheat belly', shrink sufficiently to allow you to dust off the 'skinny jeans' you saved in the back of the closet or comfortably wear the several-sizes-smaller dress or trousers from 20 years earlier.

We choose to liberate ourselves from all things wheat, while also rejecting the processed gluten-free foods made with junk carbohydrate ingredients (cornflour, rice flour, potato flour, tapioca flour), as well as processed foods (which nearly *all* contain wheat).

Though we can relearn many important dietary lessons by simply recalling many of the habits of our grandparents or great-grandparents, most of us have no desire to return to the 2, 3, 4 or more hours of preparation that were often required to prepare a full meal in their day. Thus, the quick, 30-minute or less, wheat-free effort you're now holding in your hands.

'Giving Up Wheat and Junk Carbs Is Too Hard!'

Or I might hear that it is too time-consuming, or too inconvenient, or involves too many hard-to-find ingredients.

No question: there is a period of adjustment required. After all, we creatures of the early 21st century have allowed, both purposely and inadvertently, modern wheat to balloon to 20 per cent of all the calories we eat. For some people, it can be as high as 50 per cent of calories, given the convenience, portability, ubiquity and *addictive properties* of this creation of genetics research called 'wheat'. Banning it from your diet and that of your family means an abrupt break from long-standing habits. It means no longer relying on frozen dinners and delivery pizza. It means breakfast, lunch and dinner – at least at first – need to be rethought, planned out until new habits are established, with the right mix of ingredients stocked in your store cupboards and refrigerator, and even new sources located to purchase ingredients. There is indeed an up-front investment in time and effort.

But neither do you want to devote all of your time to making this conversion.

This was the motivation for the *Wheat Belly 30-Minute (or Less!) Cookbook,* a collection of tools and ideas to help you compress the time required to navigate this new enlightened lifestyle. While we lack the convenience (with all the health compromises) of microwaving a frozen dinner in 3 minutes, or the grab-and-run appeal of a Pop-Tart, we can adopt a number of important methods to reduce the time commitment required to adhere to this unique but enormously effective approach.

To conform to such a tight timeline, I've employed several easy, commonsense, time-saving strategies, such as having a pre-made supply of the All-Purpose Baking Mix (page 19) on hand, a blend of healthy ingredients sans wheat and junk carbohydrates that can be used to create muffins, rolls or focaccia flatbread ahead of time (on the weekend, for example), which are then stored in the refrigerator for use over the course of the week. (Healthy wheat-free products are just starting to become a commercial reality but are not yet available to most people.) You will find a wide variety of sauces, dressings and dips that can convert a simple salmon fillet, for instance, into a delicious and exotic dish with just a dash of healthy sauce created with no unhealthy ingredients. There are wheat-free compliant seasoning mixes, too – with no junk fillers, such as wheat flour, cornflour or maltodextrin – that allow you to whip up delicious, fragrant and spicy dishes with minimal effort while slashing several minutes off preparation time.

I also wander out of the 30-minute time constraint with several adventurous themed menus that collect several recipes into special occasions, such as Pub Night, Romantic Evening and New Orleans Jamboree.

The goal: to allow you and your family to enjoy all the variety, flavour and health benefits of wheatlessness without sacrificing the conveniences of modern lifestyles.

Some people are concerned that their new wheat-free diet will be more costly, as we lose the commoditized (and government-subsidized) cost advantages of modern wheat. But remember: we wheat-free folk consume 400 fewer calories per person, per day, meaning less food needs to be prepared or purchased, providing a considerable built-in advantage. A family of four can be expected to consume something like 1,600 fewer calories per day, approaching the daily caloric intake of another person. Most people following the wheat-free lifestyle who are in the habit of maintaining a shopping budget therefore report that overall food costs are either *unchanged* or modestly *lower* with the switch to wheatlessness.

If you are already a seasoned wheat-free adherent, then this new 30-minute (or less!) cookbook will add some new and easy possibilities for day-to-day meal preparation, as well as some unique ideas for special occasions. If you have come to believe that a life without wheat and other unhealthy foods has to be dull and tasteless, well, you've got some interesting, spicy and delicious surprises coming your way! You will discover re-created ethnic foods, including Moroccan, Indian, Chinese, Mexican and Italian dishes, as well as reimagined foods recast into this new wheat-free lifestyle. Pizzas, soups, sandwiches, muffins, cheesecake, barbecued pork – there are very few dishes that cannot be re-created minus all unhealthy ingredients in the 30-minute (or less!) timeline. And be sure to peruse the Snacks and Desserts section, as I believe you will encounter some delightful surprises!

For those of you new to this lifestyle, the recipes and meals featured here can help you get off to a confident and tasty start without overwhelming you in complexity or underwhelming you in taste. Yes, it will mean losing some old ingredients and gaining some new, plus a few new lessons to learn in baking, thickening and ingredient choice. But reinvigorated health, potentially minus several health conditions, as well as several inches off your waist without the pull of appetite are your reward for your effort.

All right, let's get started. In the first chapter, I will discuss how several conveniences will be used in your wheat-free lifestyle to compress preparation time down to the desired 30-minute (or less!) timeline.

PUTTING TOGETHER YOUR WHEAT-FREE KITCHEN

START YOUR NEW wheat-free adventure by purging your shelves of all wheat and wheat-containing products. This is necessary to reduce the temptation to eat those chocolate-covered biscuits you've been saving and other goodies that can – even as the tiniest morsel – undo *everything* you've accomplished. It also minimizes the potential for future reexposures that can result in anything from gastrointestinal distress (bloating, cramps, diarrhoea) to joint pain, asthma and even emotional effects.

Next, you will need to do some shopping for wheat-free replacement ingredients. Your wheat-free life, for instance, will require some new flours to allow you to create sandwiches, biscuits and other baked goods using healthy non-wheat ingredients. And, for efficiency, especially to create dishes in a 30-minute timeline, a few new kitchen tools will be helpful. All in all, converting your kitchen to one that dispenses wonderfully healthy, tasty and quick wheat-free dishes really just requires some adjustments to your previous wheat-filled life.

This book serves as a guide for everyone who wishes to eliminate wheat and gluten from their lives. Wheat elimination is *not* just for the coeliac sufferer or the gluten-sensitive; it's for *everyone*. However, the advice and recipes here are indeed appropriate for the coeliac sufferer and gluten-sensitive, though additional efforts will need to be made to accomplish meticulous gluten avoidance, especially looking for 'gluten-free' on the label to avoid potential for cross-contamination.

But, before I get started on what you need to conduct your new life of wheatlessness, you first should . . .

Clean Your Kitchen!

Remember: Wheat products contain gliadin, which degrades in the gastrointestinal tract to a collection of opiates that bind to the opiate receptors of the brain. They don't cause euphoria or pain relief; they trigger appetite. Freeing yourself from the relentless appetite-stimulating effects of wheat, the frequent and intrusive thoughts of food and the increased but unnecessary calorie intake all add up to a powerful way to control impulse, weight and health.

Start by clearing your store cupboards of obvious wheat sources, such as bread, muffins, bagels, pittas, rolls, biscuits, energy bars and pastries. Don't forget the bag of wheat flour too: you will *never* need it.

After clearing the obvious wheat sources, clear the not-so-obvious sources. Examine the labels of *all* processed foods to see whether wheat in any form is found on the list of ingredients. See 'Wheat . . . by Any Other Name!' on page 13 for a list of hidden sources of wheat – yes, it's long!

Common processed foods that contain wheat include:

- Biscuits
- Breadcrumbs, panko
- Breakfast cereals
- Cookies
- Crackers
- Crips, pretzels and other snacks
- Frozen dinners
- Frozen waffles and pancakes
- Granola bars

- Ice cream, frozen yogurt
- Instant soup mixes
- Pastas
- Powdered soup mixes
- Salad dressings – bottles/dry mixes
- Sauce mixes
- Sausages, processed meats
- Seasoning mixes
- Soy sauce, teriyaki sauce

- Sweets

- Tinned soups

Get rid of it all! Remember: the gliadin protein of wheat is powerfully addictive and will pull you back into its clutches. Don't let that happen!

Restocking the Shelves
with Healthy Wheat-Free Foods

Once you've banished all wheat-containing foods from your kitchen, it will be time to restock with healthy replacements. Here are some basic ground rules to follow.

- Read labels. Look for 'wheat', 'wheat flour', 'gluten', 'vital wheat gluten', 'modified food starch', 'caramel colouring' or any of the other dozens of buzwords for concealed wheat that manufacturers slip in. Refer to 'Wheat . . . by Any Other Name!' on page 13 if you're unsure about a product. People with coeliac disease and gluten sensitivity definitely need to do this, but this is also a good practice for everyone to minimize exposure and especially to avoid the gastrointestinal and appetite-stimulating effects of wheat.

- Buy *single-ingredient natural foods* found in the produce aisle, from the butcher and at farmers' markets that don't require labels. There are no labels, for instance, on tomatoes, mushrooms, avocados, eggs or salmon.

- Avoid processed foods with multiple ingredients. A salad dressing you make yourself with olive oil, vinegar and herbs is far safer than a premixed bottled dressing with 15 ingredients.

- Lose the breakfast cereal habit. There is no such thing as a healthy breakfast cereal (at least not yet). They are land mines for wheat, not to mention other junk ingredients such as corn, sugar, high-fructose corn syrup and additives.

- Never buy a processed or prepared food unless you can view the ingredient list. Processed meats at the deli, for instance, are frequent sources of unexpected wheat exposure. Ask to see the label. If you cannot, pass it by.

- Don't even bother with the bread aisle or bakery. There's *nothing* there you need!

- Avoid prepared foods made from minced meats, such as meatballs, as these nearly always contain breadcrumbs.

- Ignore all claims of 'heart healthy', 'low fat', 'low in cholesterol', 'part of a balanced diet', etc. These claims are there for one reason: to persuade shoppers that an unhealthy food might have some health benefit. Rarely is that true. In fact, most 'heart-healthy' foods *cause* heart disease!

- Get to know your local shops, farmers' markets, health food shops and anyone else selling foods in your area. To make healthy wheat-free foods, you may need some ingredients that are not sold at all mainstream outlets. Prices also vary widely, so it helps to shop around and not be stuck with high prices for your everyday wheat-free ingredients.

Most of us who are trying to avoid wheat but are not among the most gluten-sensitive just need to look for foods and ingredients that do not list wheat or wheat-derived ingredients, while anyone with coeliac disease or extreme gluten sensitivity will require an explicit 'gluten-free' designation on the label. For instance, with dark chocolate chips, the most gluten-sensitive people will need to purchase a brand actually designated 'gluten-free', meaning it contains no wheat and no gluten and has no potential for cross-contamination from other foods and facilities. Those of us avoiding wheat but without coeliac disease or extreme gluten sensitivity can do fine with brands that are not labelled 'gluten-free' but do not list any wheat or gluten equivalents in the ingredients.

Alternative Flours

When we remove wheat, we remove the primary staple for creating breads and other baked foods. We therefore require alternative ground nuts and seeds and flours to re-create baked goods, but we must choose them carefully to avoid adding other problem ingredients. Recall that we also reject the typical replacement flours used in the gluten-free world: cornflour, rice flour, potato flour and tapioca flour, due to their extravagant capacity to send blood sugar levels through the roof.

The flours and ground nuts and seeds that we choose must be:

- Wheat-free

- Gluten-free if coeliac disease or gluten sensitivity is present

- Free of conventional gluten-free junk carbohydrate ingredients – no cornflour, potato flour, tapioca flour or rice flour

- Low in carbohydrate exposure; otherwise, we'll have high blood sugar levels and other undesirable phenomena. The dried, pulverized starch in flours can be especially destructive because the fine consistency increases surface area for digestion exponentially, resulting in rapid breakdown to blood sugar. So we need to strictly limit our exposure to carbohydrates in powdered form. The more good fats, protein and fibre the better!

- Otherwise healthy; we don't, therefore, replace a problem – wheat – with another problem

Our choices of ground nuts and seeds and flours include:

Chickpea flour	Ground pecans
Coconut flour	Ground psyllium seeds
Ground almonds and flour	Ground pumpkin seeds
Ground chia seeds and flour	Ground sesame seeds
Ground golden flaxseeds	Ground sunflower seeds
Gound hazelnuts	Ground walnuts

Note: As commonly used, 'ground' refers to the end product of grinding *whole* nuts, including skins; 'flour' refers to the end product of grinding *blanched* nuts with their skins removed, and sometimes with oils pressed out, yielding a finer flour texture and finer end result with baking.

(continued on page 8)

Important Reminders for the Gluten-Sensitive

People with coeliac disease or equivalents, such as neurological impairment or dermatitis herpetiformis, and those with gluten sensitivity need to be meticulous in avoiding wheat, gluten and non-wheat gluten sources such as barley, rye, triticale, bulgur and oats. (Not all gluten-sensitive people have gluten reactions to the avenin protein in oats, but oatmeal and oat bran skyrocket your blood sugar anyway. So kiss it goodbye and you'll be better off. You will also avoid the common cross-contamination problems of oats, which are typically prepared in facilities that handle wheat products.) Not only is meticulous gluten avoidance necessary to avoid such things as violent bowel reactions, but it is important to avoid the manyfold higher risk of gastrointestinal cancers and progressive neurological impairment that comes from even occasional exposure.

So, unlike most of us non-gluten-sensitive folk who may experience 'only' a bout of diarrhoea, mental 'fog' and fatigue or hand pain for several days, genuinely gluten-sensitive people can experience dire long-term consequences and should make every possible effort to avoid exposures, purposeful or inadvertent.

Here are some important strategies to keep in mind above and beyond just avoiding wheat and gluten.

- Getting *everyone* in the house to give up wheat and gluten really helps make life easier. It reduces exposure to tempting foods, and it reduces the potential for contamination. Don't forget that your dog, cat or other pet should also be consuming wheat- and gluten-free foods; dishing out their food is otherwise a potential exposure.

- If getting everyone else in the house to give up wheat and gluten is not possible, a diplomatic but firm segregation of foods, utensils and cooking surfaces will be necessary. (The most extreme gluten-sensitive individuals cannot tolerate this compromise, however.) Separate pots and pans, serving tools, even plates, glasses and utensils are necessary for many people.

- Help educate others that being wheat- and gluten-free is not just some food neurosis. It is how you manage *a disease condition,* just as someone with cancer requires chemotherapy. *Never* feel guilty about having to inform others about your needs.

- In a household in which there is segregation of foods and utensils, label foods so that you know which container of hummus, for instance, has had wheat-containing pitta crisps dipped into it. All it takes is someone dipping a knife into a jar of peanut butter after first buttering a slice of bread with it. Suddenly, the peanut butter that you thought was confidently gluten-free has now been contaminated and could trigger a disaster. Avoid sharing foods such as butter, nut butters, jams, cream cheese, dips and spreads, since the knife or food that contacts them may be contaminated.

- Eating outside the home is especially hazardous. Thankfully, some of the more progressive restaurants truly understand the concept of gluten cross-contamination, a trend that will spread, given the rapidly growing interest in eating wheat- and gluten-free. A meal at a restaurant where they forget and cook your food in a pan previously used to sauté breaded fish is all it takes to go down the wheat reexposure path. Adhere to this simple rule: If in doubt, don't.

- If you choose to take your chances at a restaurant, be especially careful to avoid breaded meats, foods fried in oils also used to fry breadcrumb-coated foods or other wheat-containing foods, gravies, salad dressings and most desserts. The most extremely gluten-sensitive, however, should not take even these risks.

- Check the label or check with the manufacturer of every prescription drug or nutritional supplement you take and make sure it is gluten-free.

- With rare exceptions, avoid fast-food restaurants. Sure, the salad may be gluten free and the salad dressing, too, but cross-contamination from buns and cookies prepared just a few feet away, or from using incompletely cleansed equipment, is all it takes to invite an exposure. Cross-contamination is the hurdle that many restaurants, fast-food and otherwise, have struggled with and the reason why many are reluctant to declare any of their dishes gluten-free.

- Be aware that gluten exposure can come via vehicles besides foods, including drugs, nutritional supplements, lipstick, chewing gum, shampoos, creams and cosmetics. Wheat-containing shampoo, for instance, can often be the explanation for a persistent rash. If in doubt, check with the manufacturer, but don't be surprised if the answer you get is the usual corporate-speak and/or a disclaimer that they cannot guarantee something is gluten-free because of potential cross-contamination.

- Cross-contamination can occur even in single-ingredient foods during preparation, packaging or display, such as a salad bar or food bar, or slicing meat with the same knife used to cut a sandwich.

All foods and ingredients in your kitchen, from refrigerator to pantry, should be gluten-free also, meaning not containing wheat or gluten sources – such as barley, rye, bulgur, triticale and oats – and prepared in facilities that do not handle wheat or gluten products, so there is no potential for cross-contamination. These products will have 'gluten-free' posted prominently on the package. But please, please, please remember: many gluten-free foods are just junk carbohydrates in disguise, so be selective.

Let's face it: We live in a world dominated by this thing called wheat. Inadvertent exposures *will* occur. You can only do your best to keep exposures to an absolute minimum.

The following non-wheat grains and flours are excluded.

Rye, barley, oats, triticale and bulgur are avoided due to immune cross-reactivity with wheat gluten.

Amaranth, teff, millet, chestnut, buckwheat and quinoa are off the list because of excessive carbohydrate exposure (except when limiting carbohydrate exposure may not be as important, as in snacks or desserts for kids).

Cornflour, rice flour, potato flour and tapioca flour – the typical gluten-free flours – are also off-limits, as mentioned earlier.

All flours should be stored in the refrigerator or freezer in an airtight container to slow oxidation. Alternatively, buy your nuts and seeds whole and grind them as you need them. A food processor, a high-quality food chopper (my little KitchenAid food chopper is worth its weight in gold!), or a coffee grinder all work, grinding a batch of whole nuts or seeds down within 30 to 60 seconds. Grind only to a meal or flour consistency, as grinding further will yield nut or seed butters.

Combine flours to modify the texture of the eventual end product. For instance, in the All-Purpose Baking Mix (page 19), the primary flour is ground almonds/flour, but with added coconut flour, ground golden flaxseeds and a bit of psyllium seed – a combination that works better for most purposes than ground almonds/flour alone.

Anyone with allergies to ground nuts can find several potential replacement flour sources in this list, such as coconut flour and seed flours. However, note that, if you substitute, say, coconut and sesame seed flour for ground almonds/flour in a recipe, some adjustment of liquid quantity and cooking time may be required.

Friendly Oils

Corollary to our rejection of the 'healthy whole grain' message is our dismissal of the need to limit total fat, saturated fat and cholesterol. In fact, we *add* fats and oils to our foods for their health benefits. Oils that were previously thought to be unhealthy, such as coconut oil due to saturated fat content, now make a return in this healthy, wheat-free lifestyle. Among the best oils to choose are:

- Avocado oil
- Coconut oil
- Extra-light olive oil
- Extra-virgin olive oil
- Flaxseed oil
- Organic butter and ghee
- Walnut oil

We also don't trim the fat off of our poultry, beef, pork or fish and don't skim the gelatine and fat off our soup or stock. Lard is perfectly consistent with this lifestyle, but is tough to find in a non-hydrogenated form.

Sweeteners: What You Need to Know

There are several non- or minimally nutritive sweeteners that have proven to be relatively benign and are compatible with the *Wheat Belly 30-Minute (or Less!) Cookbook* programme: stevia, erythritol, xylitol, luo han guo (monk fruit) and sucralose. These sweeteners allow you to re-create cookies, muffins and other goodies without the adverse health effects of sugar, nor the unhealthy implications of some not-so-benign sweeteners, such as aspartame.

The sugar alcohols outside of erythritol and xylitol – such as mannitol, sorbitol and maltitol – generate substantial gas, cramps and diarrhoea, not to mention increased blood sugar, and are therefore not recommended since most of us don't relish the prospect of diarrhoea with dessert.

Combining sweeteners is an especially useful strategy. If, for example, you are among those who experience the bitter aftertaste of stevia, combine stevia with, say, erythritol or luo han guo; less stevia will be required and the aftertaste will be reduced or eliminated.

Stevia

Look for pure liquid stevia, pure powdered stevia or powdered stevia with inulin; avoid stevia with maltodextrin, which is often used to bulk up stevia so that it matches the volume of sugar, cup for cup.

Erythritol

Erythritol is one of the sweeteners in Truvía (with rebiana, an isolate of stevia) and Swerve (with inulin). Avoid Pure Via, as it contains glucose and/or maltodextrin.

Xylitol

Xylitol is the most sugarlike of the chosen sweeteners: unlike the others, it yields good glazing and streusel effects. Use it only in limited quantities, however, because it has a modest capacity to raise blood sugar. And dog owners should know that xylitol can be toxic to dogs.

Luo Han Guo/Monk Fruit

Monk fruit, a natural sweetener, is rapidly becoming a favourite because it lacks the bitter aftertaste that some people experience with stevia. Like stevia, it does not raise blood sugar or cause tooth decay, lacking the adverse health effects of conventional sweeteners. It's tough to find but becoming easier as demand increases. Avoid both Monk Fruit in the Raw and Nectresse because these products contain glucose and/or maltodextrin. Be sure to read packages and look for new products coming to supermarkets that contain just monk fruit or monk fruit and erythritol.

Sucralose

There is some uncertainty about the health implications of sucralose (a potential for allergy and idiosyncratic reactions; detrimental effects on bowel flora, at least in animal studies). It is also tough to obtain as pure sucralose without maltodextrin. (Splenda is sucralose with maltodextrin.) So this is the last choice among the sweeteners.

Your Shopping List

In addition to the real, single-ingredient foods that will become the focus of your diet, such as green peppers, onions and other vegetables, as well as beef, pork, lamb, fish, chicken and other meats, the following are common ingredients needed to follow the wheat-free lifestyle. This list includes just about everything you will need to make the meals in this cookbook.

Almond milk, unsweetened

Baking powder (aluminium-free)

Cauliflower

Cheeses

Chia seeds, ground or whole

Chocolate – 100% chocolate, 85% cocoa or greater

Chocolate chips, dark

Cocoa powder, unsweetened

Coconut, shredded and unsweetened; coconut flakes

Coconut flour

Coconut milk – tinned for thickening recipes; carton for drinking

Courgettes

Cream of tartar

Dried fruit, unsweetened

Eggs

Extracts – natural almond, coconut, peppermint and vanilla

Flaxseeds, preferably ground golden

Ground almonds/flour

Ground nuts – ground almonds, hazelnuts, pecans, walnuts

Nut and seed butters – almond butter, peanut butter, sunflower seed butter

Nuts – raw almonds, Brazil nuts, hazelnuts, pecans, pistachios, walnuts; chopped pecans or walnuts for baking

Oils – avocado, coconut, extra-light olive, extra-virgin olive, flaxseed, walnut

Seeds – chia, raw pumpkin, raw sunflower and sesame

Shirataki noodles (in the refrigerated section)

Spaghetti squash

Sweeteners – liquid stevia, powdered stevia (pure or with inulin, not maltodextrin), powdered erythritol, Truvía, xylitol, luo han guo/monk fruit

Replacement Ingredients for Other Food Sensitivities

A growing number of people have food sensitivities, allergic and otherwise, that make food choices tricky. While some, if not most, food sensitivities improve or disappear when wheat is removed from the diet (probably due to loss of the gliadin small bowel permeability effect), some people do indeed need to continue to avoid the source of their sensitivities.

Here is a starting list to identify potential replacement ingredients.

Replacement Ingredients for Other Food Sensitivities

If you are sensitive to:	Consider replacing with:
Almonds	Chia seeds, chickpea flour, ground pecans, ground pumpkin seeds, ground sesame seeds, ground sunflower seeds, ground walnuts
Butter	Avocado oil, coconut oil, extra-light olive oil, ghee (unless extremely dairy-sensitive), walnut oil
Eggs	Apple purée, chia seeds, coconut milk (tinned variety), Greek yoghurt (unsweetened), ground golden flaxseeds, pumpkin purée, tofu (from non-GMO soya)
Milk	Almond milk, coconut milk (carton variety), goat milk, hemp milk, soya milk (from non-GMO soya)
Nuts	Chia seeds, pumpkin seeds, sesame seeds, sunflower seeds
Peanut butter	Almond butter, hazelnut butter, sunflower seed butter
Soured cream	Coconut milk (tinned variety)

Wheat . . . by Any Other Name!

Wheat is included in an astounding number of processed foods – because it stimulates appetite! Yes, those nice processed food manufacturers have had your number for many years. So recognizing the many varied names used for wheat products in food is essential to avoid inadvertent exposures.

It may be listed by obvious wheat labels, such as 'wheat flour', 'refined white flour', or 'vital wheat gluten'. Those are easy to spot. Consult this list for the not-so-obvious hidden sources that need to be watched out for too. They include:

Baguette

Barley

Beignet

Bran

Brioche

Bulgur

Burrito

Caramel colouring

Couscous

Crepe

Croutons

Durum

Einkorn

Emmer

Farina

Farro

Focaccia

Fu (gluten in Asian foods)

Gluten

Gnocchi

Graham flour

Gravy

Hydrolysed vegetable protein

Hydrolysed wheat starch

Kamut

Matzo

Modified food starch

Orzo

Panko (a breadcrumb mixture used in Japanese cooking)

Ramen

Roux (wheat-based sauce or thickener)

Rusk

Rye

Seitan (nearly pure gluten used in place of meat)

Semolina

Soba (mostly buckwheat but usually also includes wheat)

Spelt

Strudel

Tabbouleh

Tart

Textured vegetable protein

Triticale

Triticum

Udon

Wheat bran

Wheat germ

Wraps

Don't commit this list to memory; simply reading through it will help you to recognize the varied ways wheat can infiltrate your food. Consult this list whenever uncertainty arises.

Kitchen Tools

None of the kitchen tools listed below are absolutely essential to get started on your wheat-free lifestyle – but they sure can simplify the process and save you a lot of time! I advise just getting started with your recipes, then add gadgets as the need arises.

For instance, spiral slicers make exquisite noodle replacements out of courgettes more consistently and more quickly than doing it with a knife. If you find you or your family really likes courgette noodles, then it would be wise to invest in a Spiralizer or Spirelli device. Likewise, because I have yet to see a truly healthy ice cream in supermarket refrigerators, I offer a homemade version (page 211); a modern electric ice-cream maker is therefore a huge time- and effort-saver.

Among the most useful devices:

Electric hand mixer

Food chopper/food processor – If you're in the market for one that is inexpensive and easy to use and clean up, the KitchenAid food chopper is my favourite for around $35/£23.

Ice-cream maker

Muffin cases (paper or silicone)

Muffin tin

Spiral slicer (Spiralizer or Spirelli)

Tortilla press – Making a batch of tortillas to store for later use is much easier with this pressing device.

Waffle maker

Whoopie tin – Making perfect saucer-shaped whoopies or buns is much easier with these tins.

Wooden cocktail sticks

Ready, Set, Go!

If you've gotten this far, then you are well equipped to get started on your 30-minute wheat-free cooking adventure!

Note that, in addition to the single-dish recipes in the next several chapters, you will find an assortment of themed menus in the back of this book. I predict that you will discover just how rich, delicious, satisfying and healthy this new wheat-free lifestyle can be!

MAKING THE WHEAT-FREE LIFESTYLE AS EASY AS 1, 2, 3!

FROM THE PERSPECTIVE of health and the way you feel, the wheat-free lifestyle blows away everything I have ever seen in my lifetime. Remove a dietary poison and appetite, health and weight are transformed. The list of advantages gained by this wheat-free lifestyle ranges from head to toe, brain to bowels, appetite to sexual drive.

But there is one *disadvantage:* because we have chosen to reject this common foodstuff, this creation of genetic manipulations, an ingredient in virtually all processed foods on supermarket shelves, we lose the *convenience* of prepared foods. We can no longer buy loaves of bread, bagels by the dozen, pre-made pastry cases, just-add-milk pancake mixes or microwave-for-3-minute frozen dinners. For many people, those conveniences are a *big* part of their former diets.

Losing the convenience of processed foods means that we have to spend more time and effort creating basic foods, such as breads and salad dressings, from scratch. To economize on time and effort, however, I've created a number of mixes for baked goods, seasonings, and sauces and dressings. Once you've stocked up on these basic requirements, putting together quick meals becomes a snap.

Baking Mixes

Here are the basic recipes for mixes to make baked goods that are best prepared beforehand, then stored in the refrigerator for later use. For example, make up a batch of focaccia on the weekend, and then store it in the refrigerator to use for sandwiches over the course of the week.

Carb Watchers

All recipes in this cookbook were developed to be quick as well as to be strictly wheat-free. They were also designed to be healthy and to keep carbohydrate exposure low. Most of the recipes therefore provide a net carbohydrate content of no more than 15 grams per serving. Net carbohydrates are a very helpful idea conceived by the late low-carb guru, Dr Robert Atkins, and are calculated by subtracting fibre from total carbohydrates, since fibre has virtually no glycaemic potential:

Net carbohydrates = Total carbohydrates – Fibre

(There are some exceptions in the recipes that go just a bit higher in net carbohydrate exposure, especially some of the kid-friendly choices, since children are less susceptible to carbohydrate excesses than are adults. But none go substantially higher.)

All recipes, in addition to being wheat-free, are also free of other grains, contain little to no added sugars, use sugar and carbohydrate sources such as fruit sparingly, and likewise use starchy legumes as sparingly as possible.

ALL-PURPOSE BAKING MIX

PREP TIME: 5 MINUTES | **TOTAL TIME:** 5 MINUTES

Makes 575g (1lb 4oz)

This mix is meant to be useful for creating a variety of different bread and baked goods recipes: loaf breads, flatbreads, rolls, scones, muffins and cookies. Keeping a supply of this mix on hand will help save time in creating many of the 30-minute (or less!) meals.

400g (14oz) ground almonds/flour

130g (4½oz) ground golden flaxseeds

30g (1oz) coconut flour

2 tsp bicarbonate of soda

1 tsp ground psyllium seeds (optional)

In a large bowl, whisk together the ground almonds/flour, flaxseeds, coconut flour, bicarbonate of soda and psyllium seeds (if desired). Store in an airtight container, preferably in the refrigerator.

PER 1 TBSP: 40 calories, 2g protein, 2g carbohydrates, 3g total fat, 0g saturated fat, 1g fibre, 33mg sodium

These restrictions are more important for adults (as opposed to growing children) who are trying to facilitate weight loss, trying to correct abnormal metabolic patterns such as high blood sugar or high triglycerides or are just interested in maximizing the likelihood of ideal health.

In this cookbook, we also make use of the most benign sweeteners: stevia, monk fruit (luo han guo), erythritol and xylitol. None have implications for tooth decay; none raise blood sugar when consumed in the modest quantities used in these recipes. Because there are substantial differences among these sweeteners (especially stevia preparations) from brand to brand, we did not specify any sweetener beyond saying, for instance, sweetener equivalent to 115g (4oz) sugar. This allows you to choose your favourite sweetener. It also means that the nutritional information for the carbohydrates contained in erythritol and xylitol are not listed in the nutritional information for each recipe, though, because of the minimal to no glycaemic potential of these specific sugar alcohols, they act more like zero glycaemic index sweeteners.

SANDWICH BREAD

PREP TIME: 5 MINUTES | **TOTAL TIME:** 45 MINUTES

Makes 1 loaf (16 slices)

This sandwich bread is one of the few recipes that fall outside of our 30-minute timeline, but if made ahead of time, it will allow you to create sandwiches and other dishes within that time limit.

345g (12oz) All-Purpose Baking Mix (page 19)

1 tsp aluminium-free baking powder

½ tsp sea salt

5 eggs, separate

4 tbsp butter or coconut oil, melted

1 tbsp buttermilk or coconut milk (tinned or carton variety)

Preheat the oven to 180°C/350°F/Gas mark 4. Grease a 22 x 12cm (8½ x 4½in) loaf tin.

In a food processor, combine the baking mix, baking powder and salt. Pulse until well blended. Add the egg yolks, butter or coconut oil and buttermilk or coconut milk. Pulse until blended.

In a large bowl and using an electric mixer on high speed, beat the egg whites until soft peaks form. Pour into the flour mixture and pulse until the egg whites are evenly distributed, but do not run the machine at a constant speed. Spread into the tin and bake for 40 minutes, or until a wooden cocktail stick inserted in the centre comes out clean.

PER SLICE: 174 calories, 7g protein, 6g carbohydrates, 15g total fat, 4g saturated fat, 3g fibre, 234mg sodium

BASIC FOCACCIA

PREP TIME: 5 MINUTES | **TOTAL TIME:** 25 MINUTES

Makes 6 servings

One of the challenges of wheat-free baking with healthy substitute flours is generating vigorous 'rise' in loaf-style breads, given the lack of yeast. In our Basic Focaccia, we work around this limitation by making a flatbread – about as foolproof as a wheat-free bread gets.

This basic recipe is easily modified to create numerous variations. For example, add 2 teaspsoons ground or crushed rosemary, 1 teaspoon dried oregano and 1 teaspoon dried garlic for Italian-style flatbread. Or, after baking, brush the top with extra-virgin olive oil and sprinkle with grated Parmesan cheese. For bread that goes perfectly with cream cheese, add 1 teaspoon cinnamon and ½ teaspoon nutmeg and your choice of sweetener equivalent to 1 teaspoon sugar.

Note that the sequence of adding the ingredients specified below must be followed as written to avoid the common 'baker's ammonia' effect, the result of the bicarbonate of soda in the baking mix reacting with the proteins in the eggs, generating an ammonia smell, which is unpleasant. When you add the vinegar first, the acetic acid in the vinegar will react with the bicarbonate of soda, preventing the reaction with the egg.

230g (8oz) All-Purpose Baking Mix (page 19)

2 tbsp extra-virgin olive oil

2 tbsp vinegar

50ml (2fl oz) water

1 tsp xanthan gum (optional)

½ tsp sea salt

3 eggs, whisked

Preheat the oven to 190°C/375°F/Gas mark 5. Grease a large rimmed baking sheet.

In a large bowl, place the baking mix. In a small bowl or cup, combine the oil, vinegar, water, xanthan gum (if desired) and salt. Add to the baking mix and quickly mix together. Let sit for 1 minute, then add the whisked eggs and mix together thoroughly.

With moistened hands, place the dough on the baking sheet and shape into a 20 x 30cm (8 x 12in) rectangle.

Bake for 15 minutes, or until lightly browned. With a pizza cutter or knife, cut into six 8 x 10cm (3 x 4in) pieces. Store in the refrigerator.

PER SERVING: 289 calories, 11g protein, 10g carbohydrates, 25g total fat, 3g saturated fat, 6g fibre, 415mg sodium

HERBED FOCACCIA

PREP TIME: 15 MINUTES | **TOTAL TIME:** 35 MINUTES

Makes 6 servings

This flatbread proved a favourite among readers of my previous cookbook, providing a delicious way to enjoy ham and cheese sandwiches, smoked turkey sandwiches or a wonderful bread to dip into extra-virgin olive oil. So I brought it back with some minor changes for the 30-minute experience.

Note that the sequence of adding the ingredients specified below must be followed as written to avoid the occasional 'baker's ammonia' effect, the result of the bicarbonate of soda in the baking mix reacting with the proteins in the eggs, generating an ammonia smell, which is unpleasant. When you add the vinegar first, the acetic acid in the vinegar will react with the bicarbonate of soda, preventing the reaction with the egg.

150g (5oz) grated mozzarella or other cheese

345g (12oz) All-Purpose Baking Mix (page 19)

1 tsp xanthan gum

1 tsp aluminium-free baking powder

1¼ tsp sea salt, divided

1 tsp onion powder

½ tsp garlic powder

1½ tsp dried rosemary, crushed

1½ tsp dried oregano

80g (3oz) pitted black olives or Kalamata olives, chopped or finely sliced

40g (1½oz) sun-dried tomatoes, finely sliced

6 tbsp extra-virgin olive oil, divided

2 tbsp white vinegar or apple cider vinegar

2 eggs, separated

Preheat the oven to 190°C/375°F/Gas mark 5. Grease a baking sheet.

In a food chopper or food processor, pulse the cheese until reduced to small granules, about the size of couscous.

In a medium bowl, combine the processed cheese, baking mix, xanthan gum, baking powder, 1 teaspoon of the salt, the onion powder, garlic powder, rosemary, oregano, olives and tomatoes. Mix well. Add 2 tablespoons of the oil and the vinegar and mix quickly. Set aside.

In a large bowl and using an electric mixer on high speed, beat the egg whites until stiff. Blend in the egg yolks and 2 tablespoons of the remaining oil at low speed. Pour into the reserved dough mixture and mix together with a spoon.

Place the dough onto the baking sheet and, using your hands, shape into a 28 x 30cm (11 x 12in) rectangle. Alternately, cover the dough with parchment paper and use a rolling pin to roll the dough 1cm (½in) thick.

Bake for 10 minutes. Remove from the oven and, using the blunt handle of a wooden spoon or other small rounded instrument, make small depressions in the surface every couple of centimetres or so. Brush the surface with the remaining 2 tablespoons oil and sprinkle with the remaining ¼ teaspoon salt. Bake for 8 minutes, or until lightly browned.

Use a pizza cutter or knife to cut the flatbread into six 10 x 15cm (4 x 6in) slices.

PER SERVING: 545 calories, 19g protein, 19g carbohydrates, 47g total fat, 7g saturated fat, 11g fibre, 905mg sodium

BASIC SANDWICH MUFFINS

PREP TIME: 5 MINUTES | **TOTAL TIME:** 20 MINUTES

Makes 4 halves or 2 complete

Put egg and sausage between 2 of these sandwich muffin halves and you have a breakfast muffin. Or use them for a mini hamburger.

To save time on busy days, make the muffins ahead of time. The recipe can, of course, be doubled or tripled to make larger batches. For delicious flavoured muffins, add ¼ teaspoon each dried rosemary and dried oregano.

115g (4oz) All-Purpose Baking Mix (page 19)

½ tsp aluminium-free baking powder

½ tsp sea salt

2 tbsp extra-virgin olive oil

1 egg

1 tbsp water + additional water if needed

Preheat the oven to 180°C/350°F/Gas mark 4. Grease 4 cups of a whoopie tin.

In a bowl, combine the baking mix, baking powder and salt. Stir in the oil thoroughly. Add the egg and stir until mixed. If the dough is too stiff, add the water 1 tablespoon at a time.

Divide the dough among the 4 whoopie cups. Using a spoon, flatten the mounds until approximately 1cm (½in) thick, leaving a shallow well in the centre. Bake for 12 minutes, or until the edges begin to brown. Allow to cool for 3 minutes before carefully removing from the tin.

PER SERVING (½ MUFFIN): 240 calories, 8g protein, 8g carbohydrates, 21g total fat, 2g saturated fat, 5g fibre, 417mg sodium

FLAXSEED WRAP BAKING MIX

PREP TIME: 5 MINUTES | **TOTAL TIME:** 5 MINUTES

Makes 280g (10oz)

Ground golden flaxseeds make a wonderful wrap that can replace its wheat- or corn-equivalent in any recipe.

260g (9oz) ground golden flaxseeds

1 tsp aluminium-free
    baking powder

1½ tsp onion powder

1 tsp garlic powder

½ tsp sea salt

In a medium bowl, whisk together the flaxseeds, baking powder, onion powder, garlic powder and salt. Store in an airtight container, preferably in the refrigerator.

PER 35G (1¼OZ) SERVING: 123 calories, 6g protein, 9g carbohydrates, 9g total fat, 0g saturated fat, 8g fibre, 149mg sodium

FLAXSEED WRAP

PREP TIME: 5 MINUTES | **TOTAL TIME:** 15 MINUTES

Makes 1

Here's one more workhorse recipe I've brought back from the original book. It has proven to be a perennial favourite, though this time made from our Flaxseed Wrap Baking Mix (page 25).

35g (1¼oz) Flaxseed Wrap Baking Mix
(page 25)

1 tsp coconut oil, melted, or olive oil

1 egg

1 tbsp water

In a medium bowl, combine the baking mix, oil, egg and water until a thin, pourable dough forms.

Grease a microwaveable 23cm (9in) glass or plastic pie plate. Pour the dough into the plate, using a spatula to empty the bowl. Tilt the plate to coat the bottom uniformly. Microwave on high power for 2–3 minutes, or until cooked. Let cool for 5 minutes. (Alternatively, bake in a greased ovenproof pie plate at 190°C/375°F/Gas mark 5 for 10 minutes, or until the centre is cooked.)

To remove the tortilla, lift up an edge with a spatula. If it sticks, use a pancake turner to gently loosen from the plate. Turn the wrap over and top with desired ingredients or store in the refrigerator for later use.

PER SERVING (1 WRAP): 234 calories, 12g protein, 9g carbohydrates, 18g total fat, 6g saturated fat, 8g fibre, 220mg sodium

PITTA CRISPS

PREP TIME: 5 MINUTES | **TOTAL TIME:** 5 MINUTES

Makes 1 serving

By simply microwaving the ingredients for the Flaxseed Wrap a bit longer, you can easily create a bowl of crispy pitta-like crisps that can be dipped into fresh Guacamole (page 32) or Spicy Hummus (page 33). If you want more crisps, work with 2 pie plates. That way, you can mix up a batch of batter while another batch cooks in the microwave.

35g (1¼oz) Flaxseed Wrap Baking Mix (page 25)

1 tsp coconut oil, melted, or olive oil

1 egg

1 tbsp water

In a medium bowl, combine the baking mix, oil, egg and water until a thin, pourable dough forms.

Grease a microwaveable 23cm (9in) glass or plastic pie plate. Pour the dough into the plate, using a spatula to empty the bowl. Tilt the plate to coat the bottom uniformly. Microwave on high power for 3½–5 minutes, or until crispy. Break apart by hand into desired shape and size.

PER SERVING: 234 calories, 12g protein, 9g carbohydrates, 18g total fat, 6g saturated fat, 8g fibre, 220mg sodium

TORTILLA BAKING MIX

PREP TIME: 5 MINUTES | **TOTAL TIME:** 5 MINUTES

Makes 540g (1lb 3oz)

This basic mix is suited to making up a batch of tortillas. Whip up, for example, 4 tortillas, and you will have enough to last almost a week in the refrigerator. You can quickly slap together a quesadilla or mini-pizza in a few minutes just by keeping some of these around and piling on a few ingredients.

390g (14oz) ground golden flaxseeds

100g (3½oz) ground almonds/flour

2 tbsp onion powder

2 tsp garlic powder

1½ tsp sea salt

In a large bowl, whisk together the flaxseeds, ground almonds/flour, onion powder, garlic powder and salt. Store in an airtight container, preferably in the refrigerator.

PER 30G (1¼OZ) SERVING: 126 calories, 6g protein, 8g carbohydrates, 10g total fat, 0g saturated fat, 7g fibre, 142mg sodium

TORTILLAS

PREP TIME: 5 MINUTES | **TOTAL TIME:** 10 MINUTES

Makes 4

Here's how we put the Tortilla Baking Mix to work to yield 4 tortillas per batch.

125g (4½oz) Tortilla Baking Mix   2 eggs

Preheat the oven to 190°C/375°F/Gas mark 5. Line a large baking sheet with parchment paper.

Pour the baking mix into a large bowl. Whisk in the eggs until combined. Divide the dough into 4 equal portions.

Roll each ball between 2 pieces of parchment paper until it is 15cm (6in) in diameter. Alternatively (and much easier!), use a tortilla press lined with parchment paper.

Place on the baking sheet, with both pieces of parchment, and bake for 5 minutes, or until golden.

Store in the refrigerator.

PER SERVING (1 TORTILLA): 162 calories, 9g protein, 8g carbohydrates, 12g total fat, 1g saturated fat, 7g fibre, 177mg sodium

Sauces and Dressings

It happens with seasoning mixes, and it happens all too often with shop-bought sauces and dressings: hidden wheat or other unhealthy ingredients. One common ingredient, for instance, in many salad dressings, virtually all barbecue sauces, ketchup and other condiments, is high-fructose corn syrup. In fact, a quick examination of the labels at your local supermarket will show that there are very rare examples of truly healthy sauces and dressings!

So here is a collection of healthy, wheat-free, junk ingredient–free sauces and dressings that can help make interesting and delicious 30-minute (or less!) dishes!

BASIL PESTO

PREP TIME: 5 MINUTES | **TOTAL TIME:** 5 MINUTES

Makes 195g (7oz)

I love growing my own basil plants and then picking the lushest leaves and grinding them into this fresh pesto, which bursts with the magical combination of olive oil, Parmesan cheese and the basil. For especially delightful but simply elegant dishes, pour this on top of some shirataki noodles with an extra dash of sea salt and pepper, or add a couple of tablespoons to scrambled eggs (yes, the colour is wacky, but it's delicious!).

50g (2oz) fresh basil

2 tbsp pine nuts

2 garlic cloves, chopped

75ml (3fl oz) extra-virgin olive oil

25g (1oz) Parmesan cheese, grated

¼ tsp sea salt

1½ tsp white balsamic vinegar

In a food chopper or food processor, combine the basil, pine nuts and garlic. Chop or process into a paste. Add the oil, cheese, salt and vinegar and chop or process until the ingredients are blended and the pesto is bright green.

PER 1 TBSP: 86 calories, 1g protein, 1g carbohydrates, 9g total fat, 1.5g saturated fat, 0g fibre, 70mg sodium

GUACAMOLE

PREP TIME: 10 MINUTES | **TOTAL TIME:** 10 MINUTES

Makes 6 servings

Here's something to dip your Pitta Crisps (page 27) into, or to spread on a wrap, tortilla or sandwich. Guacamole is a satisfying and delicious dip for raw veggies, too.

3 ripe avocados, halved, pitted and peeled

1 onion, coarsely chopped

1 serrano chilli, coarsely chopped (wear plastic gloves when handling)

2 garlic cloves, coarsely chopped

10g (⅓oz) fresh coriander, finely chopped

Juice of 1 lime

½ tsp sea salt

1 tomato, coarsely chopped

In a food chopper or food processor, combine the avocados, onion, chilli, garlic, coriander, lime juice and salt. Chop or pulse until slightly chunky and combined. Add the tomato and pulse until the desired consistency.

PER SERVING: 129 calories, 2g protein, 9g carbohydrates, 11g total fat, 1g saturated fat, 5g fibre, 140mg sodium

SPICY HUMMUS

PREP TIME: 10 MINUTES | **TOTAL TIME:** 10 MINUTES

Makes 615g (1lb 6oz)

Hummus is such a versatile dip and sandwich spread that I thought it would be best to provide a homemade, do-it-yourself version. It's also less costly making it yourself, rather than purchasing the deli version, which can get pretty pricey.

For a deeper, more mellow flavour, try roasting the garlic. Simply cut off and discard the top 1cm (½in) of a whole garlic bulb, drizzle with ½ teaspoon olive oil and wrap in foil. Bake in a 190°C/375°F/Gas mark 5 oven for 40–45 minutes, or until the cloves are soft. Allow to cool for 20 minutes before squeezing the soft garlic cloves into the chickpea mixture.

If you don't like the taste of tahini, you can substitute toasted sesame oil or leave it out altogether.

50ml (2fl oz) extra-virgin olive oil

1 tin (425g/15oz) chickpeas, rinsed and drained

3–4 garlic cloves, finely chopped

3 tbsp lemon juice

2 tbsp tahini

½ tsp cayenne pepper (optional)

½ tsp paprika

½ tsp sea salt

1 tbsp grated Pecorino or Parmesan cheese (optional)

1 tbsp pine nuts (optional)

1 tbsp chopped chives (optional)

In a food chopper or food processor, pulse the olive oil, chickpeas and garlic. Add the lemon juice, tahini, cayenne pepper (if desired), paprika and salt and process until thoroughly mixed and smooth. Sprinkle with the cheese, pine nuts or chives, if desired. Store in an airtight container in the refrigerator.

PER 90G (3OZ) SERVING: 118 calories, 3g protein, 6g carbohydrates, 10g total fat, 1g saturated fat, 1g fibre, 179mg sodium

TOMATO SAUCE

PREP TIME: 10 MINUTES | **TOTAL TIME:** 30 MINUTES

Makes 1.75 litres (3 pints)

As with other sauces and dressings, many shop-bought tomato sauces contain added sugar or high-fructose corn syrup. The challenge in making it ourselves is keeping the time required down to our 30-minute maximum. Adding red wine to the sauce takes off the residual bitterness that ordinarily requires 2 hours of simmering on the stove to reduce. I keep a bottle of Côtes du Rhône, Burgundy or Cabernet Sauvignon that has been open a bit too long to be drinkable, in the refrigerator for uses such as this.

2 tbsp extra-virgin olive oil

2 shallots or 1 medium onion, finely chopped

3 garlic cloves, finely chopped

1 tsp crushed red chillies

4 tins (400g/14oz each) chopped tomatoes

170g (6oz) tomato purée

2 tbsp Italian Seasoning Mix* (page 56)

Sweetener equivalent to 1 tbsp sugar

Sea salt and pepper to taste

50ml (2fl oz) red wine

In a large saucepan over a medium heat, heat the olive oil until hot. Cook the shallots, garlic and crushed chillies until the shallots are translucent.

Meanwhile, pour the tomatoes into a blender and blend until you reach the desired consistency (the briefer the blending, the chunkier the sauce). Transfer the tomatoes to the saucepan. Stir in the tomato purée, seasoning mix, sweetener, salt and pepper. Bring to a simmer over a medium heat. Reduce the heat to low and simmer, stirring occasionally, for 20 minutes. Stir in the red wine and remove from the heat.

*Or substitute 2 tsp dried basil, 2 tsp dried oregano, 2 tsp dried rosemary.

PER 125ML (4½FL OZ) SERVING: 74 calories, 2g protein, 11g carbohydrates, 2g total fat, 0g saturated fat, 2g fibre, 261mg sodium

BARBECUE SAUCE

PREP TIME: 5 MINUTES | **TOTAL TIME:** 25 MINUTES

Makes 940g (2lb 1oz)

This variation on the perennial sauce favourite for meat fits perfectly into the wheat-free lifestyle. Slather it on ribs, steaks, pork or fish for added spice and pizzazz.

3 garlic cloves, finely chopped

1 tbsp chilli powder

1 tbsp olive oil

800g (1¾lb) tomato passata

2 tbsp black treacle

1 tbsp apple cider vinegar

2 tbsp mustard

½ tsp cayenne pepper

½ tsp sea salt

1 tbsp onion powder

Sweetener equivalent to 55g (2oz) sugar

In a medium saucepan over a medium heat, cook the garlic and chilli powder in the oil for 3 minutes. Add the tomato passata, black treacle, vinegar, mustard, cayenne pepper, salt, onion powder and sweetener. Bring to a boil, reduce the heat to low, cover, and simmer for 15 minutes, stirring occasionally. Remove from the heat and cool before storing in the refrigerator.

PER 80G (3OZ) SERVING: 47 calories, 1g protein, 9g carbohydrates, 1g total fat, 0g saturated fat, 1g fibre, 316mg sodium

THAI RED CURRY SAUCE

PREP TIME: 5 MINUTES | **TOTAL TIME:** 5 MINUTES

Makes 435g (15oz)

Convert just about any meat or vegetable into a spicy, flavourful dish just by adding this Thai Red Curry Sauce.

1 tin (400ml/14fl oz) coconut milk

2 tbsp red curry paste

¾ tsp rice vinegar

¾ tsp tamari

In a small bowl, combine the coconut milk, curry paste, vinegar and tamari. Stir until well mixed. Store in an airtight container in the refrigerator.

PER 145G (5OZ) SERVING: 269 calories, 3g protein, 6g carbohydrates, 27g total fat, 24g saturated fat, 2g fibre, 477mg sodium

GINGER-MISO SAUCE

PREP TIME: 5 MINUTES | **TOTAL TIME:** 5 MINUTES

Makes 165g (6oz)

Here's an Asian spin on a sauce that can be used as a marinade or sauce for chicken or fish, as a unique alternative for barbecued ribs, or just as a salad dressing. Find miso paste in natural health food or Asian food shops.

1½ tbsp miso paste

2 tbsp sesame oil

1 tbsp rice vinegar

1 tsp wasabi powder (optional)

1 tsp crushed fresh ginger

½ tsp crushed garlic
    (1 small clove)

1 tsp onion powder

2 tbsp sesame seeds

50 ml (2fl oz) water

In a small bowl, whisk together the miso, sesame oil, vinegar, wasabi (if desired), ginger, garlic, onion powder, sesame seeds and water until the miso is dissolved. Store in an airtight container in the refrigerator.

PER 1 TBSP: 50 calories, 1g protein, 1g carbohydrates, 5g total fat, 0.5g saturated fat, 0g fibre, 144mg sodium

DILLED CUCUMBER YOGHURT SAUCE

PREP TIME: 10 MINUTES | **TOTAL TIME:** 10 MINUTES

Makes 395g (14oz)

This easy sauce makes a delicious accompaniment to Middle Eastern Lamb Burgers (page 146).

250g (9oz) whole milk plain Greek yoghurt

90g (3oz) peeled, grated cucumber

2 tbsp extra-virgin olive oil

1 tbsp finely chopped fresh dill

1 tsp finely chopped fresh mint

¼ tsp garlic powder

½ tsp kosher salt

⅛ tsp freshly ground black pepper

In a small bowl, combine the yoghurt, cucumber, oil, dill, mint, garlic powder, salt and pepper. Stir well.

PER 100G (3½OZ) SERVING: 99 calories, 6g protein, 3g carbohydrates, 7g total fat, 1g saturated fat, 0g fibre, 242mg sodium

TARTAR SAUCE

PREP TIME: 5 MINUTES | **TOTAL TIME:** 5 MINUTES

Makes 190g (6½oz)

Simple and traditional, this version of Tartar Sauce is truly healthy!

125g (4½oz) olive oil mayonnaise

50g (2oz) finely diced pickled dill cucumbers

1 tsp dried onions

2 tsp lemon juice

In a small bowl, stir together the mayonnaise, pickle, dried onions and lemon juice. Serve with fish.

PER 2 TBSP: 69 calories, 0g protein, 1g carbohydrates, 7g total fat, 1g saturated fat, 0g fibre, 230 mg sodium

MAYONNAISE

PREP TIME: 5 MINUTES | **TOTAL TIME:** 10 MINUTES

Makes about 575g (1lb 4oz)

Yes: mayonnaise.

More and more people have come to me saying, 'I don't trust the shop-bought mayonnaise and all its peculiar ingredients. How do I make my own with healthy ingredients?'

Well, here you go!

All ingredients should be at room temperature. If any ingredients are cool or refrigerated, soak them in hot water until they're at room temperature before proceeding with the recipe. You can also add flavourings, such as paprika or dill, to the finished mayo.

3 egg yolks

2 tsp Dijon mustard

¼ tsp sea salt

450ml (16fl oz) extra-light olive oil

50ml (2fl oz) white wine vinegar

In a food processor or with an electric mixer, combine the yolks, mustard and salt. Pulse or blend at high speed. Slowly pour in the oil over several minutes and process or blend until the mixture thickens. Add the vinegar and process until combined.

Store in an airtight container in the refrigerator for up to 1 week.

PER 1 TBSP: 102 calories, 0g protein, 0g carbohydrates, 12g total fat, 2g saturated fat, 0g fibre, 26mg sodium

GARLICKY MAYO SPREAD

PREP TIME: 5 MINUTES | **TOTAL TIME:** 5 MINUTES

Makes about 275g (10oz)

Use this zesty spread on wheat-free sandwiches or to top the Salmon Croquettes (page 173).

255g (9oz) Mayonnaise
(page 40)

1 tbsp lemon juice

1 garlic clove, finely chopped

⅛ tsp sea salt

⅛ tsp freshly ground black pepper

In a small bowl, combine the mayonnaise, lemon juice, garlic, salt and pepper. Stir until well blended. Store in an airtight container in the refrigerator.

PER 1 TBSP: 101 calories, 0g protein, 0g carbohydrates, 11g total fat, 1.5g saturated fat, 0g fibre, 102mg sodium

SPICY CAJUN MAYO

PREP TIME: 5 MINUTES | **TOTAL TIME:** 5 MINUTES

Makes 140g (5oz)

This flavourful mayo can serve as a spicy topping for sandwiches or wraps or as a unique dip for veggies. You can also add it to egg yolks to make quick but unique devilled eggs.

125g (4½oz) Mayonnaise (page 40)

1 tsp tomato purée

1 tsp lemon juice

¾ tsp Cajun Seasoning Mix (page 58)

In a small bowl, combine the mayonnaise, lemon juice, tomato purée and seasoning mix. Stir well.

PER 1 TBSP: 103 calories, 0g protein, 0g carbohydrates, 12g total fat, 2g saturated fat, 0g fibre, 36mg sodium

JAPANESE CARROT-GINGER DRESSING

PREP TIME: 10 MINUTES | **TOTAL TIME:** 10 MINUTES

Makes about 500ml (18fl oz)

If you've ever had a green salad at a Japanese restaurant, the salad leaves themselves are not generally too impressive . . . but that carrot-ginger dressing? Wow! Well, here it is, re-created for you to enjoy on your salads at home.

You can do better than the iceberg lettuce typically used in Japanese restaurants. Instead, pair this dressing with varieties such as romaine. Rocket is especially delicious with this dressing.

3 large carrots, sliced

2 tbsp coarsely chopped fresh ginger

1 shallot, coarsely chopped

120ml (4fl oz) extra-light olive oil or coconut oil

1 tbsp toasted sesame oil

50ml (2fl oz) rice vinegar

2 tbsp water

1 tbsp gluten-free soy sauce or miso paste

In a food processor or blender, combine the carrots, ginger, shallot, olive oil or coconut oil, sesame oil, vinegar, water and soy sauce or miso paste. Pulse until reduced to a thin paste. Store in an airtight container in the refrigerator.

PER 2 TBSP: 80 calories, 0g protein, 3g carbohydrates, 8g total fat, 1g saturated fat, 1g fibre, 127mg sodium

HERBED RANCH DRESSING

PREP TIME: 5 MINUTES | **TOTAL TIME:** 5 MINUTES

Makes 500ml (18fl oz)

Shop-bought mayonnaise is used in this recipe to simplify preparation. However, the quality of this ranch dressing will depend on the quality of the mayonnaise you choose. So be sure to choose brands that have no unhealthy ingredients, such as hydrogenated oils, or make your own (page 40). Thankfully, most mayonnaises are a simple combination of oils, eggs, vinegar and seasonings. The oil used is usually the omega-6-rich soybean oil, but if you shop around, you can find brands made with olive oil and coconut oil. Alternatively, use conventional mayonnaise but replace one-third with your choice of healthy oil.

250g (9oz) mayonnaise

110ml (4fl oz) soured cream

110ml (4fl oz) buttermilk

2 tbsp lemon juice

5g (¼oz) parsley, chopped

2 tbsp chopped chives

¼ tsp dried dill

In a medium bowl, combine the mayonnaise, soured cream, buttermilk, lemon juice, parsley, chives and dill. Mix well. Pour into a bottle or jar and store in the refrigerator.

PER 2 TBSP: 117 calories, 1g protein, 1g carbohydrates, 12g total fat, 2g saturated fat, 0g fibre, 103mg sodium

RANCH DRESSING

PREP TIME: 5 MINUTES | **TOTAL TIME:** 5 MINUTES

Makes about 450ml (16fl oz)

Back by popular demand, this ranch dressing recipe was included in the first two books. It has proven such a hit that I include it here, too.

225ml (8fl oz) soured cream

125g (4oz) mayonnaise

50g (2oz) Parmesan cheese, grated

1 tsp garlic powder

1½ tsp onion powder

1 tbsp distilled white vinegar

Pinch of sea salt

1–2 tbsp water

In a medium bowl, whisk together the soured cream, mayonnaise, cheese, garlic powder, onion powder, vinegar, salt and 1 tablespoon of the water. If you prefer a thinner consistency, add the additional 1 tablespoon water. Pour into a bottle or jar and store in the refrigerator.

PER 2 TBSP: 53 calories, 1g protein, 2g carbohydrates, 5g total fat, 2g saturated fat, 0g fibre, 104mg sodium

CREAMY PESTO DRESSING

PREP TIME: 5 MINUTES | **TOTAL TIME:** 5 MINUTES

Makes 150ml (5fl oz)

This makes a great spread for sandwiches, as well as a dressing for green salads.

50ml (2fl oz) soured cream

50ml (2fl oz) buttermilk

3 tbsp prepared Basil Pesto (page 31)

1 tbsp grated Pecorino cheese

In a small bowl, combine the soured cream, buttermilk, pesto and cheese. Mix well. Pour into a bottle or jar and store in the refrigerator.

PER 2 TSP: 25 calories, 1g protein, 1g carbohydrates, 2g total fat, 1g saturated fat, 0g fibre, 27mg sodium

CREAMY TOMATO-CORIANDER DRESSING

PREP TIME: 5 MINUTES | **TOTAL TIME:** 5 MINUTES

Makes 440ml (15½fl oz)

This is a slightly different variation of traditional Thousand Island dressing. Like Thousand Island, it is also useful on sandwiches.

250g (9oz) mayonnaise

125g (4½oz) tomato sauce

2 tbsp chopped sun-dried tomatoes

1 tbsp apple cider vinegar

20g (¾oz) coriander, chopped

¼ tsp freshly ground black pepper

¼ tsp sea salt

In a small bowl, combine the mayonnaise, tomato sauce, sun-dried tomatoes, vinegar, coriander, pepper and salt. Stir until thoroughly mixed. Pour into a bottle or jar and store in the refrigerator.

PER 2 TBSP: 141 calories, 1g protein, 2g carbohydrates, 15g total fat, 2g saturated fat, 1g fibre, 244mg sodium

MOROCCAN DRESSING

PREP TIME: 5 MINUTES | **TOTAL TIME:** 5 MINUTES

Makes 350ml (12fl oz)

The unique combination of spices in the Moroccan Seasoning Mix also makes a great salad dressing. Mediterranean salads with romaine lettuce, Kalamata olives and feta cheese go especially well with this dressing.

225ml (8fl oz) extra-virgin olive oil

110ml (4fl oz) vinegar (red wine, white wine or apple cider)

4 tsp Moroccan Seasoning Mix (page 55)

Combine the oil, vinegar and seasoning mix in a cruet or jar. Shake until mixed. Store in the refrigerator.

PER 1 TBSP: 87 calories, 0g protein, 0g carbohydrates, 9g total fat, 1.5g saturated fat, 0g fibre, 0mg sodium

SPICY ITALIAN DRESSING

PREP TIME: 5 MINUTES | **TOTAL TIME:** 5 MINUTES

Makes 350ml (12fl oz)

Once you make a batch of the Italian Seasoning Mix, there's no reason not to have a bottle of homemade Spicy Italian Dressing on hand, too!

225ml (8fl oz) extra-virgin olive oil

110ml (4fl oz) vinegar (red wine, white wine, balsamic or white balsamic)

1 tbsp Italian Seasoning Mix (page 56)

½ tsp sea salt

Combine the oil, vinegar, seasoning mix and salt in a cruet or jar. Shake until mixed. Store in the refrigerator.

PER 1 TBSP: 87 calories, 0g protein, 0g carbohydrates, 9g total fat, 1g saturated fat, 0g fibre, 49mg sodium

SUN-DRIED TOMATO ITALIAN DRESSING

PREP TIME: 5 MINUTES | **TOTAL TIME:** 5 MINUTES

Makes 400ml (14fl oz)

This is a useful all-round, everyday salad dressing.

225ml (8fl oz) extra-virgin olive oil

50ml (2fl oz) red wine vinegar

50ml (2fl oz) water

35g (1¼oz) sun-dried tomatoes
  (oil-packed), chopped

2 tsp Italian Seasoning Mix (page 56)

2 tbsp grated Pecorino cheese

In a blender, combine the oil, vinegar, water, tomatoes, seasoning mix and cheese. Blend until thoroughly mixed. Pour into a bottle or jar and store in the refrigerator.

PER 2 TSP: 55 calories, 0g protein, 0g carbohydrates, 6g total fat, 1g saturated fat, 0g fibre, 9mg sodium

PLUM-CHIA JAM

PREP TIME: 5 MINUTES | **TOTAL TIME:** 15 MINUTES

Makes about 365g (13oz)

Choose the juiciest plums when they are ripe and slightly soft and they will yield a delicious jam when combined with the gel action of chia. Spread this treat on scones, a slice of Basic Focaccia (page 21) or wheat-free pancakes.

4 plums

3 tbsp ground chia seeds

Sweetener equivalent to 55g (2oz) sugar

1 tbsp lemon juice

Stone the plums and coarsely chop. Place in a food chopper or food processor and pulse for 1 minute, or until reduced to a pulpy liquid.

In a medium bowl, combine the processed plums, chia seeds, sweetener and lemon juice. Mix well. Set aside for 10 minutes. Store in an airtight container in the refrigerator. Stir prior to serving.

PER 2 TBSP: 26 calories, 1g protein, 6g carbohydrates, 1g total fat, 0g saturated fat, 1g fibre, 0mg sodium

STRAWBERRY BUTTER

PREP TIME: 5 MINUTES | **TOTAL TIME:** 10 MINUTES

Makes 200g (7oz)

This simple embellishment to butter yields a delightful spread for a slice of Sandwich Bread (page 20). It is easily modified by replacing the strawberries with other berries, such as cranberries (raw or cooked), fresh or dried apricots or other fruit. Wrap a portion of the finished butter in clingfilm, then foil, and it will keep in the freezer for 1 month.

75g (3oz) fresh strawberries

125g (4½oz) butter, at room temperature

Sweetener equivalent to 2 tbsp sugar

In a food chopper or food processor, pulse the strawberries briefly until they are finely chopped.

In a medium bowl, combine the strawberries, butter and sweetener. Mix thoroughly. Alternatively, combine all of the ingredients in the bowl of a stand mixer and mix on low speed with the paddle attachment until thoroughly blended. Store in an airtight container in the refrigerator.

PER 1 TBSP: 107 calories, 0g protein, 2g carbohydrates, 12g total fat, 7g saturated fat, 0g fibre, 101mg sodium

HERBED BUTTER

PREP TIME: 5 MINUTES | **TOTAL TIME:** 10 MINUTES

Makes 245g (8½oz)

Keeping a bit of this fragrant herbed butter on hand helps liven up vegetables, mashed cauliflower, chicken, beef and fish with just a dollop. It can also be featured in a bowl at the table or formed (when semi-solid) into any shape desired. I like keeping a variety of herbed and flavoured butters stored in ramekins in the refrigerator. Change the herbs, if desired; chives, sage or thyme all work well. Wrap a portion of the finished butter in clingfilm, then aluminium foil, and it will keep in the freezer for 1 month.

225g (8oz) butter, at room temperature

15g (1½ oz) fresh basil, fresh rosemary or fresh marjoram, chopped

½ tsp garlic powder or 1 tsp crushed garlic

½ tsp sea salt

In a bowl, combine the butter, herbs, garlic and salt. Mix thoroughly. Alternatively, combine all the ingredients in the bowl of a stand mixer and mix on low speed with the paddle attachment until thoroughly blended. Store in an airtight container in the refrigerator.

PER 1 TBSP: 102 calories, 0g protein, 0g carbohydrates, 12g total fat, 7g saturated fat, 0g fibre, 150mg sodium

Seasoning Mixes

Yes, even prepared seasoning mixes contain wheat – and maltodextrin and cornflour and sugar and BHT (butylated hydroxytoluene) and other ingredients that add up to potential health issues . . . just from spices!

Single-ingredient herbs and spices, dried or fresh, are nearly always wheat-free and free of other undesirables. These recipes allow you to assemble your own healthy seasoning mixes that can be kept on hand to further trim time and effort off many recipes.

Many of the recipes in this book make use of these healthy seasoning mixes, untainted by unhealthy ingredients. Ideally, mix up a batch of each ahead of time to store on your shelves in an airtight container. Of course, if you find yourself going through your seasoning mixes quickly, double, triple or otherwise multiply the ingredients to generate larger batches to store.

Since the calories and carbohydrates are negligible in these mixes, no nutritional information is included.

MOROCCAN SEASONING MIX

PREP TIME: 5 MINUTES | **TOTAL TIME:** 5 MINUTES

Makes about 5 tablespoons

2 tbsp ground cumin

1 tbsp ground coriander

2 tsp ground ginger

1½ tsp ground cinnamon

1 tsp cayenne pepper

1 tsp ground cardamom

½ tsp ground cloves

1 tsp dried orange peel (optional)

In a small bowl, combine the cumin, coriander, ginger, cinnamon, cayenne pepper, cardamom, cloves and orange peel, if using. Store in an airtight container.

ITALIAN SEASONING MIX

PREP TIME: 5 MINUTES | **TOTAL TIME:** 5 MINUTES

Makes about 9 tablespoons

2 tbsp dried basil

2 tbsp dried oregano

2 tbsp dried rosemary, crushed

1 tbsp dried marjoram

1 tbsp garlic powder

1 tbsp onion powder

1 tsp freshly ground black pepper

In a small bowl, combine the basil, oregano, rosemary, marjoram, garlic powder, onion powder and pepper. Store in an airtight container.

TACO SEASONING MIX

PREP TIME: 5 MINUTES | **TOTAL TIME:** 5 MINUTES

Makes about 7 tablespoons

3 tbsp chilli powder

1½ tbsp onion powder

2 tsp paprika

2 tsp garlic powder

1½ tsp cayenne pepper

1½ tsp ground cumin

1 tsp dried oregano

In a small bowl, combine the chilli powder, onion powder, paprika, garlic powder, cayenne pepper, cumin and oregano. Store in an airtight container.

CAJUN SEASONING MIX

PREP TIME: 5 MINUTES | **TOTAL TIME:** 5 MINUTES

Makes 6 tablespoons

2 tbsp paprika

1 tbsp garlic powder

1 tbsp onion powder

2 tsp freshly ground black pepper

1½ tsp cayenne pepper

1 tsp dried oregano

1 tsp dried thyme

½ tsp sea salt

In a small bowl, combine the paprika, garlic powder, onion powder, black pepper, cayenne pepper, oregano, thyme and sea salt. Store in an airtight container.

HERBES DE PROVENCE

PREP TIME: 5 MINUTES | **TOTAL TIME:** 5 MINUTES

Makes about 6 tablespoons

1 tbsp dried savory

1 tbsp dried rosemary, crushed

1 tbsp dried thyme

1 tbsp dried basil

1 tbsp dried marjoram

1 tbsp fennel seeds

1 tsp dried tarragon

In a small bowl, combine the savory, rosemary, thyme, basil, marjoram, fennel seeds and tarragon. Store in an airtight container.

BREAKFASTS

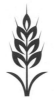

POACHED EGGS OVER ROASTED ASPARAGUS

PREP TIME: 5 MINUTES | **TOTAL TIME:** 20 MINUTES

Makes 4 servings

In order to get plenty of green vegetables over the course of the day, it sure doesn't hurt to start with breakfast. Here is a poached egg dish served over asparagus and topped with a herbed butter. Chives were chosen, but parsley, rosemary, basil and oregano – alone or in combination – also work well.

1 bunch thin asparagus (450g/1lb), tough ends removed

2 tbsp extra-virgin olive oil

½ tsp sea salt, divided

6 tbsp butter

2 tbsp finely chopped chives

1 tbsp lemon juice

2 tbsp distilled white vinegar

4 eggs

Freshly ground black pepper

Preheat the oven to 200°C/400°F/Gas mark 6. On a large rimmed baking sheet, place the asparagus in a single layer. Drizzle with the oil and sprinkle with ¼ teaspoon of the salt. Roast for 13 minutes, or until lightly browned and tender.

Meanwhile, in a small saucepan over a medium heat, melt the butter. Whisk in the chives, lemon juice and the remaining ¼ teaspoon salt. Remove from the heat and set aside.

In a large frying pan or saucepan over a medium-high heat, heat 5cm (2in) of water and the vinegar until simmering. Crack an egg into a small cup or bowl and gently slide out into the simmering water. Repeat with the remaining eggs. Simmer for 3 minutes, or until the whites are set and the yolks are slightly set but soft, or to desired doneness. An egg poacher can also be used.

Divide the asparagus evenly among 4 plates. Using a slotted spoon, carefully lift each egg out of the water, dabbing the bottom of the spoon on kitchen paper to remove any excess water, and set on a plate on top of the asparagus. Drizzle with the reserved lemon-herb butter. Season with the pepper to taste.

PER SERVING: 311 calories, 9g protein, 5g carbohydrates, 29g total fat, 14g saturated fat, 2g fibre, 422mg sodium

BACON, EGG AND TOMATO STACKS

PREP TIME: 5 MINUTES | **TOTAL TIME:** 15 MINUTES

Makes 4 servings

When you're in the mood for something a bit different from the usual scrambled or fried eggs, here is an easy 15-minute variation with tomato, Parmesan cheese and bacon.

8 rashers uncured bacon

1 large tomato, cut into four 1cm (½in) thick slices

1 tbsp extra-virgin olive oil

25g (1oz) Parmesan cheese, finely grated

4 eggs

3 tbsp distilled white vinegar

Sea salt

Freshly ground black pepper

1 tbsp snipped chives (optional)

Place the oven rack 15cm (6in) from the heat source and preheat the grill. Grease a baking sheet.

In a medium frying pan over a medium heat, cook the bacon for 5 minutes, or until the desired level of doneness. Transfer to a plate lined with kitchen paper.

Place the tomato slices in a single layer on the baking sheet. Drizzle with the oil and sprinkle each with 1 tablespoon of the cheese. Grill for 4 minutes, or until lightly browned. Set aside.

In a large frying pan or saucepan over a medium heat, heat 5cm (2in) of water and the vinegar until simmering. Crack each egg into a separate small cup or bowl. Gently add each egg, one at a time, to the simmering water. Cook for 3 to 4 minutes for soft set, 5 minutes for medium set or 7 minutes for hard set.

Place 2 slices of bacon crisscross on top of each grilled tomato. When the eggs are cooked, use a slotted spoon to carefully lift them out of the water, dabbing the bottom of the spoon on kitchen paper to remove any excess water. Place on top of the tomato and bacon stacks. Season with the salt and pepper to taste. Top with chives, if desired.

PER SERVING: 253 calories, 23g protein, 2g carbohydrates, 20g total fat, 8g saturated fat, 1g fibre, 950mg sodium

HUEVOS RANCHEROS OVER PAN-FRIED QUESO BLANCO

PREP TIME: 5 MINUTES | **TOTAL TIME:** 15 MINUTES

Makes 4 servings

Queso blanco is a firm, mild fresh cheese. Its unique quality is that it browns and softens without melting or losing shape. It should not be confused with queso fresco, which is more of a 'crumbly' fresh cheese, much like feta.

225g (8oz) queso blanco cheese,* cut into four 1cm (½in) thick slices

2 tbsp butter

4 eggs

¼ tsp sea salt

125g (4½oz) tomato salsa

1 large avocado, halved, pitted, peeled and diced

Coat a medium frying pan with olive oil cooking spray and heat over a medium-high heat. Add the cheese slices and cook for 2 minutes, or until golden brown. Turn and cook for 1 minute to brown the other side. Transfer to a plate lined with kitchen paper.

Reduce the heat to medium. Add the butter to the pan. When the butter begins to sizzle, break the eggs into the pan, and cook for 4 minutes, or until the whites are set and the yolks are the desired doneness. Season with the salt.

To assemble, place the fried eggs on top of the cheese slices. Top with the salsa and avocado.

PER SERVING: 356 calories, 19g protein, 5g carbohydrates, 30g total fat, 14g saturated fat, 2g fibre, 682mg sodium

*Note: If you can't find queso blanco, paneer would make a good alternative.

MEDITERRANEAN SCRAMBLE

PREP TIME: 10 MINUTES | **TOTAL TIME:** 20 MINUTES

Makes 4 servings

To bring out the full, rich character of this healthy Mediterranean egg dish, use free-range eggs whenever possible, the kind with orange-coloured yolks that burst with flavour.

4 tbsp extra-virgin olive oil, divided

225g (8oz) Italian sausages, thinly sliced

1 small onion, finely chopped

2 garlic cloves, finely chopped

1 tin (400g/14oz) quartered artichoke hearts, drained and chopped

35g (1¼oz) sun-dried tomatoes, finely chopped

40g (1½oz) pitted Kalamata olives, sliced

8 eggs

75g (3oz) feta cheese, crumbled

....

In a large frying pan over a medium heat, heat 2 tablespoons of the oil. Cook the sausage for 3 minutes, or until starting to brown. Add the onion and garlic and cook, stirring occasionally, for 3 minutes, or until the onion is soft and the sausage is no longer pink.

Stir in the remaining 2 tablespoons oil, the artichokes, tomatoes and olives. In a medium bowl, whisk the eggs and pour into the pan. Cook for 4 minutes, stirring occasionally, or until the eggs are set. Remove from the heat and gently stir in the cheese.

PER SERVING: 621 calories, 27g protein, 14g carbohydrates, 51g total fat, 15g saturated fat, 2g fibre, 1,467mg sodium

MINI QUICHE LORRAINES

PREP TIME: 5 MINUTES | **TOTAL TIME:** 25 MINUTES

Makes 2 servings

This is a unique interpretation of a wheat-free 'quiche', a variation of a traditional German–French dish that retains the essential flavour and feel of real cream. For a dairy-free version, you can replace the cream with coconut milk.

50g (2oz) pancetta, finely diced

2 tbsp ground almonds/flour

¼ tsp aluminium-free baking powder

2 eggs

75ml (3fl oz) cream

2 tbsp finely chopped chives or spring onion tops

⅛ tsp freshly ground black pepper

Preheat the oven to 180°C/350°F/Gas mark 4. Grease a 12-cup mini-muffin tin.

In a small frying pan over a medium heat, cook the pancetta for 5 minutes, or until lightly browned.

In a small bowl, whisk together the ground almonds/flour and baking powder. In another small bowl, combine the eggs, cream, chives or spring onion tops and pepper and beat lightly. Stir the flour mixture into the egg mixture until combined. Divide the pancetta among the muffin cups. Divide the batter evenly among the muffin cups (cups will be almost full).

Bake for 12 minutes, or until puffed and light golden. Cool for 5 minutes on a rack. Remove from the pan.

PER 6 MINI QUICHES: 351 calories, 14g protein, 3g carbohydrates, 32g total fat, 14g saturated fat, 1g fibre, 670mg sodium

CHORIZO FRITTATA

PREP TIME: 10 MINUTES | **TOTAL TIME:** 30 MINUTES

Makes 8 servings

Using chorizo sausage in this frittata saves you the effort of adding spices and flavourings – because they're already in the sausage! Combine the spice of chorizo with the healthy green of kale and you have a perfect, healthy combination that is filling. Make the frittata ahead of time, refrigerate it, and eat it over the course of the week for an entire week's worth of healthy breakfasts.

2 tbsp coconut oil

170g (6oz) chorizo sausage, chopped

1 onion, chopped

2 garlic cloves, finely chopped

225g (8oz) fresh or frozen, thawed kale, chopped

75g (3oz) sun-dried tomatoes, coarsely chopped

45g (1½oz) sliced mushrooms

10 eggs

½ tsp sea salt

Preheat the oven to 190°C/375°F/Gas mark 5.

In a large ovenproof frying pan over a medium-high heat, heat the oil. Cook the sausage, onion and garlic for 3 minutes, or until the sausage is barely pink and the onion begins to soften. Reduce the heat to medium. Stir in the kale, tomatoes and mushrooms. Cover and cook, stirring frequently, for 4 minutes, or until the mushrooms are tender.

Meanwhile, in a medium bowl, whisk the eggs and salt. Add to the pan and gently tilt to distribute the eggs. Cook for 2 minutes, or until the bottom and edges of the egg mixture become slightly firm. Transfer to the oven and bake for 10 minutes, or until the centre is nearly set.

PER SERVING: 247 calories, 15g protein, 7g carbohydrates, 18g total fat, 8g saturated fat, 1g fibre, 470mg sodium

CRAB-ASPARAGUS FRITTATA

PREP TIME: 10 MINUTES | **TOTAL TIME:** 30 MINUTES

Makes 8 servings

Here's about as nutritionally complete a breakfast as you could find! No junk breakfast cereal ingredients here: no sugar, no cornflour, no wheat – just satisfying, healthy foods that have no adverse health effects.

8 eggs

175ml (6fl oz) cream or coconut milk (tinned or carton)

10 spears asparagus, sliced diagonally into 2cm (¾in) segments

1 tin (170g/6oz) crabmeat, drained

4 tbsp extra-virgin olive oil, divided

1 small onion, finely chopped

2 garlic cloves, finely chopped

½ tsp sea salt

Preheat the oven to 190°C/375°F/Gas mark 5.

In a large bowl, whisk the eggs. Add the cream or coconut milk, asparagus, crabmeat and 2 tablespoons of the oil. Whisk to combine. Set aside.

In a large ovenproof frying pan over a medium heat, heat the remaining 2 tablespoons oil until hot. Cook the onion and garlic for 3 minutes, or until the onion is soft. Sprinkle with the salt. Pour the reserved egg mixture into the pan and stir to combine. Cook for 3 minutes, or until the edges begin to firm. Transfer to the oven and bake for 10 minutes, or until a knife inserted in the centre comes out clean.

PER SERVING: 234 calories, 10g protein, 3g carbohydrates, 20g total fat, 8g saturated fat, 1g fibre, 290mg sodium

MINI BAKED EGG CASSEROLES

PREP TIME: 5 MINUTES | **TOTAL TIME:** 25 MINUTES

Makes 4 servings

Bacon, Cheddar cheese and eggs are combined in this baked breakfast treat. If you've got some on hand, toast made with Sandwich Bread (page 20) and spread with some butter would be perfect!

8 rashers back bacon

60g (2½oz) Cheddar cheese, grated

8 eggs

2 tbsp finely chopped chives or spring onion tops (optional)

Preheat the oven to 180°C/350°F/Gas mark 4. Lightly coat 8 muffin cups with cooking spray or oil.

Line each muffin cup with 1 rasher of the back bacon. Place 1 tablespoon of the cheese in the bottom of each. Carefully break 1 egg into each muffin cup.

Bake for 15 minutes, or until just set and the whites are cooked but the yolks are still soft. Sprinkle with the chives or spring onion tops, if desired. Let stand for 5 minutes before removing from the cups and serving.

PER SERVING: 247 calories, 22g protein, 1g carbohydrates, 16g total fat, 7g saturated fat, 0g fibre, 499mg sodium

BREAKFAST CRAB CAKES

PREP TIME: 5 MINUTES | **TOTAL TIME:** 15 MINUTES

Makes 4 servings

These simple crab cakes help jazz up fried eggs, while adding the healthy nutrition of seafood to breakfast.

In place of the Italian Seasoning Mix, you can substitute ½ teaspoon dried oregano and ½ teaspoon dried basil.

1 tin (170g/6oz) crabmeat, drained	2 tsp extra-virgin olive oil
30g (1¼oz) ground golden flaxseeds	½ tsp sea salt
1 tsp Italian Seasoning Mix (page 56)	2 tbsp butter
5 eggs	

Preheat the oven to 190°C/375°F/Gas mark 5.

In a medium bowl, combine the crabmeat, flaxseeds and seasoning mix. Whisk in 1 egg, oil and salt.

Divide into four 8cm (3in) patties and place in a shallow baking pan. Bake for 10 minutes, or until cooked through and slightly firm.

Meanwhile, in a large frying pan over a medium-high heat, melt the butter. Crack the remaining 4 eggs into the pan and cook for 2 minutes, or until the whites begin to set. Turn over the eggs and cook for 2 minutes, or until the yolks are set.

Place each crab cake on a plate and top each with a fried egg.

PER SERVING: 228 calories, 17g protein, 3g carbohydrates, 17g total fat, 6g saturated fat, 2g fibre, 504mg sodium

PECAN-PUMPKIN HOTCAKES

PREP TIME: 5 MINUTES | **TOTAL TIME:** 20 MINUTES

Makes 8

Serve these fluffy, fragrant hotcakes with whipped cream, pumpkin butter or a no-sugar-added berry jam. Alongside some bacon or sausage, you've got a perfect breakfast!

1 tsp ground cinnamon

½ tsp ground nutmeg

30g (1¼oz) finely chopped pecans

Sweetener equivalent to
    55g (2oz) sugar

1 tsp bicarbonate of soda

240g (8½oz) almond butter, melted

220g (8oz) pumpkin purée

1 tsp vanilla extract

2 eggs

Preheat the oven to 180°C/350°F/Gas mark 4. Line a shallow baking tin with parchment paper.

In a large bowl, combine the cinnamon, nutmeg, pecans, sweetener and bicarbonate of soda and mix well. Stir in the almond butter, pumpkin and vanilla. In a small bowl, whisk the eggs and then stir into the mixture.

For each hotcake, scoop an eighth of the batter onto the baking tin. Bake for 12 minutes, or until slightly firm to the touch and a wooden cocktail stick inserted in the centre comes out clean.

PER HOTCAKE: 246 calories, 9g protein, 9g carbohydrates, 21g total fat, 3g saturated fat, 5g fibre, 248mg sodium

GINGERBREAD BREAKFAST CAKES

PREP TIME: 5 MINUTES | **TOTAL TIME:** 25 MINUTES

Makes 6

These cakes taste like gingerbread biscuits and will delight big and little kids: they'll feel like they're having dessert for breakfast! Minus wheat and sugar, these healthy cakes have no nutritional downside.

Spread cream cheese, butter or Plum–Chia Jam (page 51) over the top.

230g (8oz) All-Purpose Baking Mix (page 19)

1 tsp aluminium-free baking powder

1 tsp ground ginger

¾ tsp ground cinnamon

¼ tsp ground nutmeg

¼ tsp ground cloves

Sweetener equivalent to 115g (4oz) sugar

1 tsp lemon juice

50ml (2fl oz) warm water

1 tbsp black treacle

1 egg, whisked

Preheat the oven to 180°C/350°F/Gas mark 4. Line a baking sheet with parchment paper.

In a medium bowl, combine the baking mix, baking powder, ginger, cinnamon, nutmeg, cloves and sweetener and mix thoroughly.

In a small bowl, combine the lemon juice and water. Pour into the dry mixture, add the black treacle, and mix. Wait for 1 minute, and then stir in the egg.

Spoon out the dough in 6 mounds onto the baking sheet, pressing down to flatten to 2cm (¾in) thickness. Bake for 15 minutes, or until a wooden cocktail stick inserted in the centre comes out clean.

PER CAKE: 236 calories, 9g protein, 13g carbohydrates, 18g total fat, 2g saturated fat, 6g fibre, 270mg sodium

SILVER DOLLAR PANCAKES

PREP TIME: 5 MINUTES | **TOTAL TIME:** 25 MINUTES

Makes 24

These pancakes are lightly sweetened and are delicious with or without syrup.

The more fragile structure yielded by the wheat-free ground almonds/flour and coconut flour makes better small pancakes, thus the 8cm (3in) diameter suggested here.

25g (1oz) ground almonds/flour

30g (1¼oz) coconut flour

1 tsp bicarbonate of soda

Sweetener equivalent to
   1 tbsp sugar

30g (1¼oz) finely chopped walnuts

½ tsp ground cinnamon

3 eggs

135g (5oz) no-sugar-added apple purée

5 tbsp water

2 tbsp butter or coconut oil, melted or
   extra-light olive oil

In a medium bowl, whisk together the ground almonds/flour, coconut flour, bicarbonate of soda, sweetener, walnuts and cinnamon.

In a large bowl, whisk together the eggs, apple purée, water and butter or oil. Add to the flour mixture and whisk just until combined.

Lightly grease a large frying pan or griddle and heat over a medium-low heat until hot. For each 8cm (3in) pancake, pour 1 tablespoon batter onto the pan. Cook for 2 minutes, or until small bubbles form on top and the edges are cooked and lightly browned. Carefully turn and cook for 2 minutes, or until golden on the bottom. Repeat with the remaining batter.

PER 6 PANCAKES: 236 calories, 8g protein, 10g carbohydrates, 19g total fat, 6.5g saturated fat, 4g fibre, 438mg sodium

BREAKFAST CHEESECAKE

PREP TIME: 10 MINUTES | **TOTAL TIME:** 30 MINUTES + COOLING TIME

Makes 8 servings

Yes, cheesecake for breakfast! Made ahead of time, this simple and light cheesecake can be a special treat to start your morning. Because it is made with ricotta, rather than cream cheese, this Breakfast Cheesecake is lighter in texture than standard cheesecake. And it's not just for breakfast; this recipe can serve as a light dessert, too.

If desired, top with Strawberry Glaze (page 216) or Plum–Chia Jam (page 51).

250g (9oz) ricotta cheese, at room temperature

55g (2oz) coconut flour

Sweetener equivalent to 170g (6oz) sugar

4 tsp lemon juice

4 eggs, separated

1 tsp vanilla extract

Preheat the oven to 190°C/375°F/Gas mark 5. Grease a 23 x 23cm (9 x 9in) baking tin.

In a medium bowl, place the cheese, flour, sweetener, lemon juice, egg yolks and vanilla.

In another medium bowl, with an electric mixer on high speed, beat the egg whites until stiff peaks form. Using the same beaters, beat the cheese mixture until smooth. With a spoon, gently fold the egg whites into the cheese mixture until thoroughly combined.

Pour into the baking tin. Bake for 20 minutes, or until the edges begin to brown and a wooden cocktail stick inserted in the centre comes out clean. Cool slightly before serving.

PER SERVING: 122 calories, 8g protein, 5g carbohydrates, 7g total fat, 4.5g saturated fat, 3g fibre, 77mg sodium

KID-FRIENDLY

BREAKFAST BISCUITS

PREP TIME: 10 MINUTES | **TOTAL TIME:** 25 MINUTES

Makes 12 biscuits

'Breakfast' and 'biscuits' ordinarily don't belong together . . . unless we replace all of the unhealthy ingredients with healthy ingredients! Because these biscuits are mostly made of nuts, coconut, egg and apple, they are perfectly healthy and compatible with any breakfast.

I use dried apples for sweetness, which is a way to obtain just a bit of natural sweetness but with less sugar exposure than from other dried fruits, such as raisins or dates.

230g (8oz) All-Purpose Baking Mix (page 19)

1 tsp ground cinnamon

¼ tsp sea salt

Sweetener equivalent to 115g (4oz) sugar

30g (1¼oz) unsweetened coconut flakes

60g (2½oz) chopped walnuts

45g (1½oz) chopped dried apples

100ml (4fl oz) whole milk plain Greek yoghurt

2 tbsp butter, melted

1 egg

1 tsp vanilla extract

Preheat the oven to 180°C/350°F/Gas mark 4. Line a baking sheet with parchment paper.

In a large bowl, combine the baking mix, cinnamon, salt, sweetener, coconut, walnuts and dried apples.

In a small bowl, combine the yoghurt and butter. Add the egg and vanilla and mix well. Pour into the flour mixture and stir until well combined. The dough will be thick. Use a tablespoon to form balls consisting of 3 tablespoons each and place on the baking sheet. Lightly wet your hands and use your palms or a large spoon to flatten to 1cm (½in) thickness.

Bake for 13 minutes, or until golden. The biscuits will be soft. Allow to cool slightly before transferring to a rack to cool completely.

PER BISCUIT: 204 calories, 7g protein, 10g carbohydrates, 17g total fat, 4.5g saturated fat, 4g fibre, 160mg sodium

CINNAMON-PECAN SCONES

PREP TIME: 10 MINUTES | **TOTAL TIME:** 25 MINUTES + COOLING TIME

Makes 8 scones

Whip up a batch or two of these Cinnamon–Pecan Scones to eat over the course of the week for a quick, filling and healthy breakfast. Optionally, top with Plum–Chia Jam (page 51).

230g (8oz) All-Purpose Baking Mix
    (page 19)

3 tbsp coconut flour

½ tsp sea salt

1½ tsp ground cinnamon

50ml (2fl oz) coconut oil, cold

Sweetener equivalent to
    55g (2oz) sugar

30g (1¼oz) chopped pecans

50ml (2fl oz) buttermilk or tinned
    coconut milk

1 egg

Preheat the oven to 180°C/350°F/Gas mark 4. Line a baking sheet with parchment paper.

In a large bowl, combine the baking mix, coconut flour, salt and cinnamon. Using a pastry cutter, cut the oil into the flour mixture for 1 minute, or until incorporated and the mixture resembles damp sand. Stir in the sweetener, pecans, buttermilk or coconut milk and egg, mixing just until blended. The dough will be thick and stiff.

Use a tablespoon to scoop the dough and loosely shape it into 8 equal balls. Place 5cm (2in) apart on the baking sheet. Use your hands or a large spoon to lightly flatten to 1cm (½in) thickness. Bake for 13 minutes, or until lightly browned around the edges. Remove to a rack and cool for 5 minutes.

PER SCONE: 265 calories, 8g protein, 10g carbohydrates, 24g total fat, 8g saturated fat, 6g fibre, 258mg sodium

PESTO BREAKFAST SCONES

PREP TIME: 5 MINUTES | **TOTAL TIME:** 20 MINUTES

Makes 4 scones

Alongside some scrambled or fried eggs, these savoury pesto scones round out a healthy breakfast, complete with plenty of olive oil, nuts and cheese. If you don't have time to make homemade pesto, you can substitute your favourite shop-bought brand.

115g (4oz) All-Purpose Baking Mix (page 19)

55g (2oz) coconut flour

2 tbsp ground golden flaxseeds

1 tsp aluminium-free baking powder

2 tbsp grated Parmesan cheese

50ml (2fl oz) water

1 tbsp vinegar

1 egg

2–4 tbsp Basil Pesto (page 31)

Preheat the oven to 190°C/375°F/Gas mark 5. Line a baking sheet with parchment paper.

In a medium bowl, combine the baking mix, coconut flour, flaxseeds, baking powder and cheese. Stir in the water and vinegar, then allow to sit for 1 minute.

Mix in the egg and pesto, combining thoroughly. The mixture will be very stiff.

Spoon out the dough onto the baking sheet in four 2cm (¾in) thick mounds. Bake for 15 minutes, or until firm to the touch.

PER SCONE: 305 calories, 12g protein, 17g carbohydrates, 23g total fat, 5g saturated fat, 11g fibre, 369mg sodium

HERBED BISCUITS AND GRAVY

PREP TIME: 10 MINUTES | **TOTAL TIME:** 25 MINUTES

Makes 10 servings

Biscuits and gravy, the ultimate American comfort food, is re-created here with delicious gravy that you can pour over hot biscuits. Because it contains no wheat or other unhealthy thickeners, such as cornflour, there should be no blood sugar or insulin issues with this dish, nor joint pain, oedema, acid reflux, mind 'fog' or dandruff. Life is good without wheat!

While the gravy is also dairy-free for those with dairy intolerances, the biscuits are not, as they contain both cheese and butter. For dairy-free biscuits, omit the cheese and replace the butter with oil, such as coconut, extra-light olive or walnut.

<table>
<tr><td>

BISCUITS

125g (4½oz) Cheddar cheese, grated

230g (8oz) All-Purpose Baking Mix
   (page 19)

1 tsp dried basil

1 tsp dried rosemary, crushed

¾ tsp bicarbonate of soda

½ tsp sea salt

2 eggs

110ml (4fl oz) butter or coconut oil,
   melted, or extra-virgin olive oil

</td><td>

GRAVY

2 tbsp extra-virgin olive oil

450g (1lb) sausagemeat

400ml (14fl oz) beef stock

30g (1¼oz) coconut flour

50ml (2fl oz) tinned coconut milk

½ tsp onion powder

½ tsp garlic powder

½ tsp sea salt

</td></tr>
</table>

Preheat the oven to 190°C/375°F/Gas mark 5. Line a baking sheet with parchment paper

To make the biscuits: In a food chopper or food processor, pulse the cheese to a fine, granular consistency. Transfer to a large bowl and add the baking mix, basil, rosemary, bicarbonate of soda and salt. Mix thoroughly. Add the eggs and butter or oil and mix thoroughly. The dough will be thick.

Spoon out the dough onto the baking sheet in ten 10cm (4in) rounds. Bake for

10 minutes, or until lightly browned and a wooden cocktail stick inserted in the centre of a biscuit comes out clean.

To make the gravy: While the biscuits are baking, in a large frying pan over a medium heat, heat the oil. Cook the sausagemeat, breaking it up as it browns, for 8 minutes, or until no longer pink. Transfer to a plate and set aside.

Return the pan to the heat and increase to medium-high. Heat the stock until nearly boiling. Reduce the heat to medium-low. Whisk in the flour a tsp at a time, over 5 minutes (stop adding when the gravy obtains the desired thickness). Pour in the coconut milk and stir well. Add the onion powder, garlic powder and salt. Return the reserved sausage to the pan and simmer over low heat for 5 minutes. Add additional salt to taste.

Ladle the gravy onto the biscuits just before serving.

PER SERVING: 457 calories, 17g protein, 8g carbohydrates, 41g total fat, 15g saturated fat, 5g fibre, 976mg sodium

STRAWBERRY-COCONUT SCONES

PREP TIME: 10 MINUTES | **TOTAL TIME:** 30 MINUTES

Makes 20 scones

All right, I may have pushed the 30-minute time envelope here just by a bit . . . but it is so worth it! These scones are exceptionally tasty and deliciously crumbly with a streusel-like surface. Your family will surely forgive you the extra 5 or so minutes!

30g (1¼oz) ground golden flaxseeds

175ml (6fl oz) cold water

110g (4oz) coconut flour

30g (1¼ oz) shredded or desiccated
  unsweetened coconut

Sweetener equivalent to
  2 tbsp sugar

1 tsp bicarbonate of soda

¼ tsp sea salt

110g (4oz) strawberries, finely chopped

110ml (4fl oz) coconut oil, melted

1 egg

Preheat the oven to 190°C/375°F/Gas mark 5. Line a baking sheet with parchment paper.

In a small mug or bowl, combine the flaxseeds and water and stir briefly. Place in the freezer for 5 minutes.

Meanwhile, in a large bowl, combine the flour, coconut, bicarbonate of soda, salt and strawberries. Mix well. Stir in the oil and combine thoroughly.

Remove the flaxseed mixture from the freezer and whisk in the egg. Stir into the flour mixture. The dough will be somewhat stiff. Use a tablespoon to scoop the dough onto the baking sheet.

Bake for 17 minutes, or until a wooden cocktail stick inserted in the centre of a scone comes out clean.

PER SCONE: 101 calories, 2g protein, 5g carbohydrates, 9g total fat, 7g saturated fat, 3g fibre, 99mg sodium

STRAWBERRY-PEANUT BUTTER SUNDAES

PREP TIME: 10 MINUTES | **TOTAL TIME:** 10 MINUTES

Makes 4 servings

The flavour of these sundaes is reminiscent of a peanut butter and strawberry jam sandwich. They can easily be made ahead of time in portable containers and eaten on the go or packed to take along with you.

500g (1lb 2oz) whole milk plain Greek yoghurt

60g (2½oz) natural no-sugar-added peanut butter

50ml (2fl oz) cream

Sweetener equivalent to 55g (2oz) sugar

1 tsp vanilla extract

2 tbsp ground golden flaxseeds

150g (5oz) sliced strawberries

40g (1½oz) lightly salted roasted peanuts, chopped

In a medium bowl, combine the yoghurt and peanut butter, mixing until blended. Stir in the cream, sweetener, vanilla and flaxseeds and mix well. In 2 small bowls or sundae glasses, spoon one-quarter of the yoghurt mixture and top with half of the strawberries. Divide the remaining yoghurt mixture between the 2 bowls. Top with the remaining strawberries and the peanuts.

PER SERVING: 301 calories, 18g protein, 15g carbohydrates, 19g total fat, 5g saturated fat, 4g fibre, 127mg sodium

KEFIR SMOOTHIES

Each recipe yields approximately 300ml (½ pint). Kefir is a fermented milk drink that has lots of health benefits. If you can't find it, use whole milk yoghurt instead. All recipes, of course, can be doubled or tripled to make a batch that will last several days in the refrigerator.

PREP TIME: 5 MINUTES | **TOTAL TIME:** 5 MINUTES

KID-FRIENDLY

PIÑA COLADA SMOOTHIE

Makes 1 serving

A healthy breakfast or snack, the tropical flavours of this piña colada smoothie will persuade any spouse or child that the wheat-free lifestyle is every bit as interesting as a wheat-containing one! Optionally, mix in some raw pumpkin seeds, sunflower seeds or dry-roasted pistachios.

185g (6½oz) kefir or whole milk yoghurt

2 tbsp crushed unsweetened pineapple

3 tbsp shredded or desiccated unsweetened coconut

Sweetener (optional)

In a large glass, combine the kefir or yoghurt, pineapple, coconut and sweetener (if desired). Stir well.

PER SERVING: 247 calories, 8g protein, 16g carbohydrates, 17g total fat, 13g saturated fat, 3g fibre, 90mg sodium

APPLE PIE SMOOTHIE

Makes 1 serving

With all the flavours of a slice of freshly baked apple pie, this smoothie can be served as a stand-alone breakfast, as a delicious topping for vanilla ice cream or as a simple dessert.

250g (9oz) kefir or whole milk yoghurt

2 tbsp finely chopped apple

Sweetener equivalent to 2 tbsp sugar

¼ tsp ground cinnamon

¼ tsp ground nutmeg

In a large glass, combine the kefir or yoghurt, apple, sweetener, cinnamon and nutmeg. Stir well.

PER SERVING: 162 calories, 9g protein, 14g carbohydrates, 8g total fat, 5g saturated fat, 1g fibre, 113 mg sodium

CHOCOLATE-COCONUT SMOOTHIE

Makes 1 serving

If you love chocolate without coconut, just leave out the coconut. And the mint extract was added for you mint lovers, but it's optional. For extra decadence, add some mini dark chocolate chips.

250g (9oz) kefir or whole milk yoghurt

2 tbsp unsweetened shredded or desiccated coconut

2 tsp unsweetened cocoa powder

Sweetener equivalent to 2 tbsp sugar

3 drops natural peppermint extract (optional)

In a large glass, combine the kefir or yoghurt, coconut, cocoa, sweetener and peppermint extract (if desired). Stir well.

PER SERVING: 238 calories, 10g protein, 16g carbohydrates, 16g total fat, 11g saturated fat, 3g fibre, 117mg sodium

QUICK MUFFINS

Quick muffins are single-serve muffins that you make in a mug or ramekin. Because they can be made in a microwave, the entire process takes about 5 minutes, perfect for a quick, on-the-run, healthy breakfast in the morning. If desired, quick muffins can also be baked in the oven using an ovenproof ramekin. Bake at 190°C/375°F/Gas mark 5 for 25 minutes, or until a wooden cocktail stick inserted in the centre comes out clean. And, as always, taste your batter before cooking to gauge sweetness and adjust if needed.

KID-FRIENDLY

APPLE–SPICE QUICK MUFFIN

PREP TIME: 5 MINUTES | **TOTAL TIME:** 5 MINUTES

Makes 1 muffin

This basic muffin can be made spicier by adding ⅛ teaspoon cloves, finely chopped apples and more apple purée, particularly if you are not too concerned about carbohydrate exposure (such as with kids or serious athletes).

60g (2½oz) All-Purpose Baking Mix (page 19)	Sweetener equivalent to 1 tbsp sugar
¼ tsp ground cinnamon	1 egg
⅛ tsp ground nutmeg	2 tbsp unsweetened apple purée
Pinch of sea salt	1 tbsp butter, melted

In a medium bowl, combine the baking mix, cinnamon, nutmeg, salt and sweetener. Whisk in the egg. Add the apple purée and butter, and whisk thoroughly. Use a rubber spatula to scrape the mixture into a big mug or a 275g (10oz) ramekin.

Microwave on high power for 2 minutes, or until a wooden cocktail stick inserted in the centre comes out clean. Allow to cool for 5 minutes.

PER MUFFIN: 506 calories, 19g protein, 19g carbohydrates, 43g total fat, 11g saturated fat, 10g fibre, 644mg sodium

TRIPLE-BERRY QUICK MUFFIN

PREP TIME: 5 MINUTES | **TOTAL TIME:** 5 MINUTES

Makes 1 muffin

These simple, quick muffins are packed with healthy ingredients: nuts, berries and plenty of protein and good-for-you fats. For crunch, consider adding dry-roasted (unsalted) pistachios or cashew, walnut or pecan fragments.

60g (2½oz) All-Purpose Baking Mix (page 19)

¼ tsp ground cinnamon

Sweetener equivalent to 1 tbsp sugar

Pinch of sea salt

1 egg

2 tbsp milk

1 tbsp butter, melted

55g (2oz) frozen or fresh mixed berries

In a medium bowl, combine the baking mix, cinnamon, sweetener and salt. Whisk in the egg. Add the milk, butter and berries and whisk thoroughly. Use a rubber spatula to scrape the mixture into a large mug or a 275g (10oz) ramekin.

Microwave on high power for 2 minutes, or until a wooden cocktail stick inserted in the centre comes out clean. (If using fresh berries, microwave for 1½ minutes.) Allow to cool for 5 minutes.

PER MUFFIN: 526 calories, 20g protein, 21g carbohydrates, 44g total fat, 11g saturated fat, 11g fibre, 558mg sodium

COCONUT-CHOCOLATE QUICK MUFFIN

PREP TIME: 5 MINUTES | **TOTAL TIME:** 5 MINUTES

Makes 1 muffin

If a richer, though higher in carbohydrate/sugar muffin is desired (such as for the kids), add a tbsp of dark chocolate chips prior to microwaving or top with dark chocolate shavings after microwaving.

60g (2½oz) All-Purpose Baking Mix (page 19)

2 tsp unsweetened cocoa powder

1 tbsp unsweetened shredded coconut

¼ tsp ground cinnamon

Sweetener equivalent to 2 tbsp sugar

Pinch of sea salt

1 egg

2 tbsp milk

1 tbsp butter, melted

In a medium bowl, combine the baking mix, cocoa, coconut, cinnamon, sweetener and salt. Whisk in the egg. Add the milk and butter and whisk thoroughly. Use a rubber spatula to scrape the mixture into a large mug or 275g (10oz) ramekin.

Microwave on high power for 2 minutes, or until a wooden cocktail stick inserted in the centre comes out clean. Allow to cool for 5 minutes.

PER MUFFIN: 554 calories, 20g protein, 19g carbohydrates, 48g total fat, 14g saturated fat, 11g fibre, 553mg sodium

BLUEBERRY CHEESECAKE FRUIT CUPS

PREP TIME: 10 MINUTES | **TOTAL TIME:** 10 MINUTES

Makes 4 servings

Can anybody turn down blueberry cheesecake for breakfast?

Remember: in the wheat-free lifestyle, problem ingredients are replaced with healthy ingredients. This means that dishes like these simple Blueberry Cheesecake Fruit Cups can serve as a healthy breakfast.

225ml (8fl oz) double cream

225g (8oz) cream cheese, softened

Sweetener equivalent to 80g (3oz) sugar, or to taste

½ tsp lemon extract

125g (4½oz) whole milk plain Greek yoghurt

155g (5½oz) blueberries

60g (2½oz) chopped walnuts

In a chilled medium bowl, whip the cream with an electric mixer for 3 to 4 minutes, or until stiff peaks form. Set aside.

In another medium bowl using the same beaters, beat the cream cheese for 1 minute, or until creamy. Add the sweetener, lemon extract and yoghurt and beat for 1 minute, or just until blended. Gently fold in the whipped cream until well combined. Fold in the blueberries and walnuts.

Evenly divide into 4 sundae glasses or serving dishes. Serve immediately, or chill until firm, if desired.

PER SERVING: 531 calories, 12g protein, 12g carbohydrates, 51g total fat, 25g saturated fat, 2g fibre, 200mg sodium

BREAKFAST NUT MIX

PREP TIME: 10 MINUTES | **TOTAL TIME:** 20 MINUTES + COOLING TIME

Makes 1kg (2lb 3oz)

Here's your answer to breakfast cereal – but this cereal has *none* of the problems of the stuff that lines an entire aisle at your supermarket! Serve this nut mix with some coconut milk, almond milk or dairy milk, cold or hot. Top with a handful of fresh, dried or freeze-dried unsweetened pomegranate or other dried unsweetened berries per serving.

I make use of the modest fruit sugar in raisins. If you're serving the granola to your children and they prefer it sweeter, add just a bit of stevia or other sweetener. The use of raisins will allow you to minimize the use of sweetener.

30g (1¼oz) raisins

110ml (4fl oz) coconut milk

2 tbsp coconut oil, melted

1 tsp vanilla extract

½ tsp almond extract

280g (10oz) raw sunflower seeds

260g (9oz) raw pumpkin seeds

125g (4oz) raw chopped pecans

90g (3oz) raw flaked almonds

110g (4oz) unsweetened coconut flakes

Preheat the oven to 180°C/350°F/Gas mark 4.

In a food chopper or food processor, chop or pulse the raisins until reduced to a paste. Place in a small bowl and add the coconut milk and oil. Mix thoroughly. Add the vanilla and almond extract and stir to combine. Set aside.

In a large bowl, combine the sunflower seeds, pumpkin seeds, pecans, almonds and coconut. Stir in the reserved raisin mixture until well mixed.

Spread on a large baking sheet and bake for 15 minutes, stirring once, or until lightly browned. Remove and allow to cool.

PER 55G (2OZ) SERVING: 329 calories, 9g protein, 11g carbohydrates, 28g total fat, 11g saturated fat, 4g fibre, 7mg sodium

LIGHT MEALS
AND SIDE DISHES

CREAM OF MUSHROOM SOUP WITH CHIVES

PREP TIME: 10 MINUTES | **TOTAL TIME:** 30 MINUTES

Makes 8 servings

Wheat-free and dairy-free, this creamy mushroom soup makes a filling meal by itself or a substantial accompaniment to pork, chicken or beef dishes.

If dairy avoidance is not an issue for you, the olive oil can be substituted with butter and the coconut milk substituted with cream or whole milk.

2 tbsp extra-virgin olive oil

1 onion, finely chopped

2 garlic cloves, finely chopped

450g (1lb) baby portobello or button mushrooms, coarsely chopped

1 tsp sea salt, or to taste

½ tsp freshly ground black pepper

675ml (1¼ pints) chicken stock

1 tin (400ml/14fl oz) coconut milk

2 chopped fresh chives

In a large frying pan over a medium-high heat, heat the oil. Cook the onion for 3 minutes, or until soft. Add the garlic and cook for 1 minute. Add the mushrooms, salt and pepper. Reduce the heat to medium, cover, and cook for 5 minutes, or until the mushrooms are softened.

Stir in the chicken stock and coconut milk. Bring to a slow boil and simmer for 3 minutes.

Ladle or pour the mixture into a blender and blend until smooth (in batches, if necessary). Serve topped with the chives.

PER SERVING: 181 calories, 5g protein, 8g carbohydrates, 15g total fat, 10g saturated fat, 2g fibre, 338mg sodium

CURRY CAULIFLOWER SOUP

PREP TIME: 5 MINUTES | **TOTAL TIME:** 30 MINUTES

Makes 4 servings

As with most dishes in our wheat-free world, this soup is deceptively filling. This rich, thick cauliflower soup, with the flavour of curry, will warm your insides and satisfy you served by itself or with finger sandwiches, scones or a green salad.

2 tbsp extra-virgin olive oil

1 large onion, halved and sliced

1 large head cauliflower, chopped

2 tbsp curry powder

1 tsp ground cumin

¼ tsp sea salt

1 litre (1¾ pints) chicken stock, divided

225ml (8fl oz) double cream or
    tinned coconut milk

In a large saucepan over a medium-high heat, heat the oil. Add the onion and cauliflower and cook for 10 minutes, or until browned. Stir in the curry powder, cumin and salt. Cook for 1 minute. Add half the stock and bring to the boil. Reduce the heat to medium and cook, covered, for 8 minutes, or until the cauliflower is very tender.

Ladle or pour the mixture into a blender and blend until smooth (in batches, if necessary). Return to the saucepan with the cream or coconut milk and the remaining stock. Stir to combine. Cook for 5 minutes.

PER SERVING: 370 calories, 11g protein, 19g carbohydrates, 30g total fat, 15g saturated fat, 6g fibre, 618mg sodium

TOMATO AND FENNEL SOUP

PREP TIME: 5 MINUTES | **TOTAL TIME:** 25 MINUTES

Makes 4 servings

This simple soup recipe requires only a few minutes of preparation, but yields a tasty, filling accompaniment to any meat dish. Optionally, add chicken or pork by browning the meat first, then tossing it into the mix.

50ml (2fl oz) extra-virgin olive oil

1 large onion, thinly sliced

1 bulb fennel, halved, cored and thinly sliced

2 garlic cloves, finely chopped

600ml (1 pint) chicken stock

1 tin (400g/14oz) chopped tomatoes

½ tsp sea salt

In a large frying pan over a medium-high heat, heat the oil. Cook the onion, fennel and garlic for 10 minutes, or until very soft. (Reduce the heat to medium, if necessary, to keep the vegetables from overbrowning.)

Add the stock, tomatoes with their juice and salt and bring to the boil. Reduce the heat to a simmer, cover and cook for 10 minutes.

PER SERVING: 200 calories, 5g protein, 14g carbohydrates, 14g total fat, 2g saturated fat, 3g fibre, 727mg sodium

KID-FRIENDLY

EGG DROP SOUP

PREP TIME: 5 MINUTES | **TOTAL TIME:** 10 MINUTES

Makes 4 servings

This Chinese restaurant favourite is healthy and simple to re-create, though minus the unhealthy thickeners often used. This basic recipe is easily modified by adding, for instance, a tablespoon of Sriracha hot chilli sauce or some stir-fried vegetables.

1 litre (1¾ pints) chicken stock

1 tsp grated fresh ginger

1 tsp tamari or gluten-free
    soy sauce

¼ tsp sea salt

2 tsp coconut flour

2 eggs, whisked

3 spring onions, sliced diagonally

In a large saucepan, bring the stock, ginger, tamari or soy sauce and salt to a slow boil. Stir in the flour until dissolved. Turn off the heat. From approximately 20–25cm (8–10in) above the soup, slowly drizzle in the eggs while stirring the soup slowly in a circular motion. Continue to stir for approximately 30 seconds after the eggs have been poured in.

Stir in the spring onions and serve.

PER SERVING: 57 calories, 5g protein, 3g carbohydrates, 3g total fat, 1g saturated fat, 1g fibre, 1,083mg sodium

HAMBURGER SOUP

PREP TIME: 5 MINUTES | **TOTAL TIME:** 25 MINUTES

Makes 4 servings

This kid-pleaser is an easy tummy-filler, and also easy to adapt to personal taste. It can be topped with soured cream, grated Pecorino or Parmesan cheese or another grated cheese of your choosing.

2 tbsp extra-virgin olive oil

1 onion, finely chopped

2 carrots, sliced

1 green pepper, coarsely chopped

2 celery sticks, halved lengthwise and sliced

450g (1lb) minced beef

1 tsp Italian Seasoning Mix (page 56)

¼ tsp sea salt

1 litre (1¾ pints) beef stock

In a large frying pan over a medium-high heat, heat the oil. Cook the onion, carrots, pepper and celery, stirring occasionally, for 3 minutes, or until starting to soften. Add the beef and cook for 3 minutes, or until barely pink. Add the seasoning mix and salt and cook for 1 minute.

Pour in the stock and bring to a boil. Reduce the heat to medium and simmer for 10 minutes, or until the vegetables are softened.

PER SERVING: 407 calories, 26g protein, 9g carbohydrates, 30g total fat, 10g saturated fat, 2g fibre, 644mg sodium

NEW ORLEANS GUMBO

PREP TIME: 10 MINUTES | **TOTAL TIME:** 30 MINUTES

Makes 4 servings

It seems like everyone from Louisiana has a favourite recipe for gumbo. All involve various methods to thicken the roux. Here, for the sake of adhering to the 30-minute timeline, I use coconut flour rather than the traditional methods, a technique that shaves off about 15 or more minutes. This recipe can serve as the basis for any number of variations, such as substituting prawns for the chicken.

2 tbsp extra-virgin olive oil or coconut oil

450g (1lb) andouille or other smoked sausage, sliced

450g (1lb) boneless, skinless chicken breasts, cut into cubes

700ml (1¼ pints) chicken stock, divided

2–3 tbsp coconut flour

1 large onion, finely chopped

2 garlic cloves, finely chopped

1 large green pepper, chopped

1 tsp Cajun Seasoning Mix (page 58)

1 tin (400g/14oz) chopped tomatoes

In a large frying pan or saucepan over a medium-high heat, heat the oil. Cook the sausage and chicken, stirring occasionally, for 7 minutes, or until lightly browned. Reduce the heat to medium. With a slotted spoon, transfer the sausage and chicken to a bowl, leaving the liquid in the pan, and set aside.

Pour a third of the chicken stock into the frying pan or saucepan. Stir in the coconut flour, 1 tablespoon every 30 seconds, until the desired thickness is achieved.

Add the onion, garlic, pepper and seasoning mix. Cook, stirring occasionally, for 3 minutes, or until the vegetables begin to soften.

Return the reserved sausage and chicken to the frying pan or saucepan, along with the tomatoes with their juice and the remaining chicken stock. Cover and cook for 8 minutes, or until the chicken is cooked through and the vegetables are softened.

PER SERVING: 500 calories, 50g protein, 15g carbohydrates, 27g total fat, 8g saturated fat, 4g fibre, 1,540mg sodium

CREAM OF CRAB SOUP

PREP TIME: 10 MINUTES | **TOTAL TIME:** 30 MINUTES

Makes 8 servings

Here's the creamiest of cream soups, thickened the good, old-fashioned way without cornflour, wheat flour or other thickeners.

1 tbsp butter

2 shallots, finely chopped

1 small red pepper, finely chopped

75g (3oz) cream cheese, cut into cubes

1 litre (1¾ pints) double cream

½ tsp sea salt

¼ tsp freshly ground black pepper

450g (1lb) lump crabmeat

2 tbsp sherry

1 tsp Cajun Seasoning Mix (page 58)

In a medium saucepan over a medium heat, melt the butter. Cook the shallots and pepper for 5 minutes, or until tender. Add the cream cheese and stir for 1 minute, or until melted. Stir in the cream, salt and black pepper. Heat until the mixture just begins to simmer (do not boil).

Reduce the heat to medium-low and simmer for 5 minutes, stirring frequently. Stir in the crabmeat, sherry and seasoning mix and cook for 5 minutes, or until heated through.

PER SERVING: 534 calories, 17g protein, 4g carbohydrates, 50g total fat, 31g saturated fat, 0g fibre, 415mg sodium

NEW ENGLAND CLAM CHOWDER

PREP TIME: 10 MINUTES | **TOTAL TIME:** 30 MINUTES

Makes 4 servings

Here's how you make a New England Clam Chowder with no problem ingredients. Enjoy this heart-warming and delicious dish with some Pesto Breakfast Scones (page 77).

This clam chowder can be made using half whole milk, half double cream or coconut milk. The non-dairy coconut version is surprisingly tasty and rich.

350g (12oz) bacon, cut into 2–3cm (1in) pieces

1 onion, finely chopped

3 celery sticks, halved and sliced

2 tsp dried thyme

1 small head cauliflower, chopped into 1cm (½in) pieces

450ml (16fl oz) half whole milk, half double cream or tinned coconut milk

¼ tsp sea salt

1 tin (280g/10oz) clams

In a large saucepan over a medium-high heat, cook the bacon for 5 minutes, or until cooked through but not crispy. With tongs or a slotted spoon, remove the bacon, leaving the drippings, and place on a plate. Set aside.

Add the onion and celery and cook, stirring frequently, for 3 minutes, or until starting to soften. Stir in the thyme, cauliflower, half whole milk, half double cream or coconut milk and salt. Bring to a simmer. Reduce the heat to medium-low, cover, and simmer, stirring occasionally, for 15 minutes, or until the cauliflower is softened.

Add the reserved bacon and the clams with their juice. Cover and cook for 3 minutes, or until heated through.

PER SERVING: 616 calories, 27g protein, 17g carbohydrates, 50g total fat, 21g saturated fat, 3g fibre, 1,143mg sodium

TUNA–TOMATO MELTS

PREP TIME: 10 MINUTES | **TOTAL TIME:** 20 MINUTES

Makes 4 servings

While they can be eaten as lunch by themselves, or as a side dish with dinner, these Tuna–Tomato Melts also make a wonderful, healthy and filling breakfast alternative.

2 tins (150g/5oz each) wild-caught tuna, drained

125g (4½oz) Mayonnaise (page 40 or shop-bought)

1 tbsp Dijon mustard

1 celery stick, finely diced

2 spring onions, thinly sliced

125g (4½oz) Cheddar cheese, grated, divided

4 large plum tomatoes, halved lengthwise

Preheat the oven to 190°C/375°F/Gas mark 5. Lightly grease a shallow 1.5 or 2 litre (1½ or 2 quart) baking dish.

In a medium bowl, with a fork or the back of a spoon, break up the tuna into small chunks. Add the mayonnaise, mustard, celery, spring onions and half the cheese and mix until well blended.

Using a spoon, scoop out the flesh of each tomato half and discard. Fill each hollowed tomato half with the tuna mixture, mounding it slightly, and place in the baking dish.

Bake for 8 minutes, or until hot. Remove from the oven and turn the oven to the grill setting. While the grill is heating, top each tomato half with 1 tablespoon of the remaining cheese. Grill for 2 minutes, or until the cheese is melted and bubbly.

PER SERVING: 323 calories, 22g protein, 12g carbohydrates, 21g total fat, 8g saturated fat, 1g fibre, 715mg sodium

AUBERGINE CAPRESE STACKS

PREP TIME: 15 MINUTES | **TOTAL TIME:** 30 MINUTES

Makes 4 servings

Aubergine, basil, and Parmesan and mozzarella cheeses combine to make a confident main dish all by itself or a bold side dish alongside a shirataki noodle or spaghetti squash 'pasta' dish topped with tomato sauce.

1 aubergine, cut into eight 5mm (¼in) thick slices

30g (1¼oz) ground golden flaxseeds

50g (2oz) Parmesan cheese, finely grated, divided

½ tsp Italian Seasoning Mix (page 56)

½ tsp sea salt

1 egg, beaten

4 tbsp olive oil, divided

2 tomatoes, each cut into four 1cm (½in) thick slices

16 large fresh basil leaves

225g (8oz) fresh mozzarella, cut into 4 equal slices

Lightly grease a baking sheet.

In a shallow bowl or dish, combine the flaxseeds, half of the Parmesan, the seasoning mix and salt. Place the egg in another shallow bowl or dish. Dip a slice of the aubergine into the egg until both sides are moistened. Dredge in the flaxseed mixture to coat. Place the breaded aubergine on a plate. Repeat until all the slices have been coated.

In a large frying pan over a medium heat, heat 2 tablespoons of the oil until hot. Cook the aubergine, covered, for 8 minutes, turning once, or until browned on both sides and tender when pierced with a fork. If needed, add 1 tablespoon of the remaining oil during cooking. Transfer to a plate lined with kitchen paper.

Meanwhile, preheat the grill. Place the tomato slices in a single layer on the baking sheet. Drizzle with the remaining 1 tablespoon oil and sprinkle each with ½ tablespoon of the remaining Parmesan. Grill for 4 minutes, or until lightly browned. Remove and set aside.

On 4 plates, place the 4 largest aubergine slices. Top each slice with a grilled Parmesan tomato, 2 basil leaves and a mozzarella slice. Top with the remaining aubergine slices, a Parmesan tomato and 2 basil leaves.

PER SERVING: 377 calories, 21g protein, 13g carbohydrates, 29g total fat, 9g saturated fat, 7g fibre, 276mg sodium

CRAB-STUFFED DEVILLED EGGS

PREP TIME: 10 MINUTES | **TOTAL TIME:** 10 MINUTES

Makes 12

Here's a quick variation on standard devilled eggs made more interesting with the addition of crabmeat.

6 hard-boiled eggs, peeled and halved lengthwise

1 tin (170g/6oz) crabmeat, drained

75g (3oz) Mayonnaise (page 40 or shop-bought)

½ tsp celery salt

1 tbsp chopped fresh parsley

Place the egg yolks in a medium bowl. Arrange the egg whites on a serving plate.

Using a fork, mash the egg yolks. Add the crabmeat, mayonnaise and celery salt. Stir until well combined. Spoon the mixture evenly into the egg white halves.

Sprinkle the parsley over the top of each egg half.

PER EGG HALF: 91 calories, 6g protein, 0g carbohydrates, 8g total fat, 2g saturated fat, 0g fibre, 124mg sodium

WASABI DEVILLED EGGS

PREP TIME: 10 MINUTES | **TOTAL TIME:** 10 MINUTES

Makes 12

Here's a unique and simple variation on the familiar devilled egg – an Asian version with the zing of wasabi.

6 hard-boiled eggs, peeled and halved lengthwise

3 tbsp Mayonnaise (page 40 or shop-bought)

1 tsp wasabi powder

½ tsp ground ginger

½ tsp rice vinegar

Place the egg yolks in a medium bowl. Arrange the egg whites on a serving plate.

Using a fork, mash the egg yolks. Add the mayonnaise, wasabi, ginger and vinegar. Stir until well combined. Spoon or pipe the mixture evenly into the egg white halves.

PER EGG HALF: 64 calories, 3g protein, 0g carbohydrates, 5g total fat, 1g saturated fat, 0g fibre, 54mg sodium

ROAST BEEF SANDWICHES
WITH HORSERADISH MAYONNAISE

PREP TIME: 5 MINUTES | **TOTAL TIME:** 5 MINUTES

Makes 2 servings

Here is the traditional deli-style roast beef sandwich made with Sandwich Bread, slathered with a horseradish mayonnaise and combined with cheese and red onion.

60g (2½oz) Mayonnaise (page 40 or shop-bought)

2 tsp horseradish sauce

4 slices Sandwich Bread (page 20)

110g (4oz) deli-sliced roast beef

50g (2oz) sliced Emmental, provolone or Asiago cheese

¼ small red onion, very thinly sliced

In a small bowl, combine the mayonnaise and horseradish.

Spread 2 slices of bread with 1 tablespoon of the mayonnaise mixture each. Layer half of the roast beef, cheese and onion on each slice of bread. Spread the remaining mayonnaise mixture on top. Top with the remaining 2 slices of bread. If desired, microwave on high power for 20 seconds to melt the cheese.

PER SERVING: 724 calories, 33g protein, 14g carbohydrates, 63g total fat, 16g saturated fat, 7g fibre, 911mg sodium

AVOCADO–HAM SANDWICHES

PREP TIME: 5 MINUTES | **TOTAL TIME:** 5 MINUTES

Makes 2 servings

This simple sandwich presents several possibilities for unique variations just by altering the topping. Add thinly sliced tomatoes or sprouts for other easy variations. For a change of pace, you can also replace the ham with other meats – wheat free, of course!

4 slices Basic Focaccia (page 21) or Sandwich Bread (page 20)

1 avocado, halved, pitted, peeled and sliced, or 4 tbsp Guacamole (page 32)

½ small red onion, thinly sliced

110g (4oz) sliced ham

2–3 tbsp Herbed Ranch Dressing (page 44), Creamy Tomato–Coriander Dressing (page 47) or Spicy Hummus (page 33)

Top 2 slices of bread with the avocado, onion and ham. Drizzle with your choice of dressing or hummus. Top with the remaining 2 bread slices.

PER SERVING: 728 calories, 33g protein, 26g carbohydrates, 59g total fat, 8g saturated fat, 15g fibre, 1,201mg sodium

MUFFULETTA SANDWICHES

PREP TIME: 5 MINUTES | **TOTAL TIME:** 5 MINUTES

Makes 4 servings

This traditional New Orleans sandwich, dripping with olive oil and chopped olives, comes in many different versions, each with enthusiastic followers. Besides not using wheat-based bread, I depart from the usual routine by using Asiago cheese for an extra-cheesy 'kick'.

Muffuletta is customarily served on sesame seed-coated bread. So, if adhering to tradition is important to you, make your Basic Focaccia Flatbread with sesame seeds sprinkled on top.

4 slices Basic Focaccia (page 21)

4 tbsp muffuletta spread or tapenade

110g (4oz) sliced ham

50g (2oz) sliced pepperoni

50g (2oz) sliced mortadella

110g (4oz) sliced provolone or Emmental cheese

50g (2oz) sliced Asiago or Gruyère cheese

Spread 2 slices of bread with the muffuletta spread or tapenade. Top evenly with the ham, pepperoni, mortadella and cheese. Top with the remaining 2 slices of bread. Carefully slice each sandwich in half.

PER SERVING: 619 calories, 32g protein, 14g carbohydrates, 50g total fat, 14g saturated fat, 7g fibre, 1,766mg sodium

PROSCIUTTO-PROVOLONE FOCACCIA

PREP TIME: 5 MINUTES | **TOTAL TIME:** 10 MINUTES

Makes 4 servings

This unique sandwich provides a medley of Italian flavours: aged prosciutto, provolone, artichokes and sun-dried tomatoes.

4 slices Basic Focaccia (page 21) or
    Herbed Focaccia (page 22)

90g (3oz) baby spinach

50g (2oz) prosciutto

4 slices provolone or Emmental cheese

4 tinned artichoke hearts, sliced

2 tbsp Sun-Dried Tomato Italian
    Dressing (page 50) or other Italian
    dressing

Preheat the oven to 180°C/350°F/Gas mark 4.

On a baking sheet, arrange the bread slices. Top evenly with the spinach, prosciutto, cheese and artichokes. Bake for 3 minutes, or until the cheese is melted. Drizzle with the dressing.

PER SERVING: 471 calories, 24g protein, 14g carbohydrates, 38g total fat, 9g saturated fat, 7g fibre, 1,147mg sodium

PEPPERONI BREAD

PREP TIME: 10 MINUTES | **TOTAL TIME:** 30 MINUTES + COOLING TIME

Makes 8 servings

If you see the kids gobble this Pepperoni Bread down, don't be fooled: It just *looks* unhealthy! After all, this 'bread' is really just made of ground nuts, coconut, cheese, eggs and pepperoni. Serve this side dish alongside a shirataki or spaghetti squash pasta dish topped with Tomato Sauce (page 34), or just serve the bread and sauce without any pasta.

150g (5oz) grated mozzarella cheese, divided

230g (8oz) All-Purpose Baking Mix (page 19)

2 tbsp extra-virgin olive oil

2 eggs, lightly whisked

1 tsp Italian Seasoning Mix (page 56)

50g (2oz) pepperoni, thinly sliced

Preheat the oven to 180°C/350°F/Gas mark 4. Line a baking sheet with parchment paper.

In a food processor, pulse half the cheese until it's a granular consistency. In a large bowl, combine the cheese with the baking mix. Stir in the oil and eggs until thoroughly mixed. The dough will be thick but moist.

With moistened hands, spread the dough onto the baking sheet and form into a 25 x 25cm (10 x 10in) square about 1cm (½in) thick. Sprinkle the seasoning mix over the dough. Arrange the pepperoni over the dough, followed by the remaining cheese.

Using the parchment paper, carefully roll one end of the bread, like a Swiss roll, until the dough is fully rolled. (It may crack initially, but the outer layer will be intact.) Bake for 20 minutes, or until lightly browned.

Allow to cool for 5 minutes before slicing.

PER SERVING: 284 calories, 13g protein, 8g carbohydrates, 24g total fat, 4.5g saturated fat, 5g fibre, 364mg sodium

ITALIAN SAUSAGE MEATBALLS WITH RED WINE SAUCE

PREP TIME: 10 MINUTES | **TOTAL TIME:** 30 MINUTES

Makes 4 servings

These meatballs can go anywhere conventional meatballs can go: alone as a starter on top of shirataki noodles or by themselves as a casual main meal with a green salad or steamed green beans, kale, broccoli or asparagus.

Any minced meat can be substituted for the Italian sausages.

450g (1lb) Italian sausages, minced

2 tbsp ground golden flaxseeds

1 egg

½ tsp Italian Seasoning Mix (page 56)

¼ tsp sea salt

2 tbsp extra-virgin olive oil or coconut oil

2 tbsp tomato sauce

50ml (2fl oz) dry red wine

In a large bowl, combine the sausage, flaxseeds, egg, seasoning mix and salt and mix thoroughly. Form into 4cm (1½in) balls.

In a large frying pan over a medium-high heat, heat the oil. Cook the meatballs for 2 minutes, turning to brown all sides. Reduce the heat to medium-low, cover, and cook for 12 minutes, stirring frequently, or until no longer pink.

With a slotted spoon, transfer the meatballs to a serving bowl.

In the same pan over low heat, cook the tomato sauce and wine for 2 minutes, stirring to loosen any brown bits from the bottom of the pan, or until heated through. Pour over the meatballs.

PER SERVING: 503 calories, 19g protein, 3g carbohydrates, 45g total fat, 14g saturated fat, 1g fibre, 986mg sodium

OPEN-FACED CHICKEN CAPRESE FOCACCIA

PREP TIME: 5 MINUTES | **TOTAL TIME:** 20 MINUTES

Makes 4 servings

The flavours of fresh basil, mozzarella cheese and tomato that make Caprese salads a perennial favourite combine to make a delightful and quick open-faced sandwich. Optionally, drizzle a few drops of balsamic vinegar over the top when adding the basil.

4 slices Basic Focaccia (page 21)

2–3 tbsp Italian Seasoning Mix (page 56)

½ tsp sea salt

2 boneless, skinless chicken breast halves

1 large tomato, cut into 4 slices

110g (4oz) mozzarella cheese, sliced

15g (½oz) fresh basil, torn

Place the oven rack 15cm (6in) from the heat source and preheat to the grill setting. Place the focaccia on a baking sheet. Set aside. Grease a baking tin.

In a large resealable plastic bag, combine the seasoning mix and salt. Add the chicken and shake to coat.

Place the chicken in the baking tin and grill for 12 minutes, turning once, or until a thermometer inserted in the thickest portion registers 75°C (165°F) and the juices run clear. Let stand for 5 minutes. Cut into thin slices.

Divide the chicken, tomato and cheese among the focaccia. Grill for 1 minute, or until the cheese is melted. Sprinkle the basil over the top of each.

PER SERVING: 490 calories, 37g protein, 15g carbohydrates, 33g total fat, 7g saturated fat, 8g fibre, 982mg sodium

BACON AND BALSAMIC CHICKEN WRAPS

PREP TIME: 5 MINUTES | **TOTAL TIME:** 15 MINUTES

Makes 4 servings

The combination of bacon and reduced balsamic vinegar adds a wonderful dimension of flavour to this chicken wrap. Add sliced tomatoes or Guacamole (page 32) for a variation.

2 tbsp extra-virgin olive oil

1 boneless, skinless chicken breast, cut into thin strips

4 rashers thick-cut back bacon

110g (4oz) mushrooms, sliced

2 tbsp balsamic vinegar

4 Flaxseed Wraps (page 26)

100g (3½oz) shredded romaine lettuce

In a large frying pan over a medium-high heat, heat the oil. Cook the chicken, bacon and mushrooms for 8 minutes, or until the chicken is no longer pink, the bacon is cooked through and the mushrooms are golden. With a slotted spoon, transfer the chicken and bacon to a plate and set aside.

Reduce the heat to low. Add the vinegar to the mushrooms in the pan. Simmer, stirring, for 1 minute, or until the vinegar has reduced. Remove from the heat.

Lay the wraps on a work surface. Arrange the reserved chicken and bacon down the centre of each wrap. Top with the lettuce and mushroom mixture. Roll up.

PER SERVING: 394 calories, 25g protein, 12g carbohydrates, 29g total fat, 8g saturated fat, 9g fibre, 384mg sodium

AVOCADO, BACON AND EGG SANDWICHES

PREP TIME: 5 MINUTES | **TOTAL TIME:** 20 MINUTES

Makes 2 servings

The combination of Cajun spices and bacon is surprisingly mouthwatering, especially along with the cool, creamy feel of fresh avocado. Don't let the small size of these sandwiches fool you: they are wonderfully filling!

4 rashers thick-cut back bacon

2 eggs

4 slices Sandwich Bread (page 20)

¼ cup Spicy Cajun Mayo (page 42)

1 avocado, halved, pitted, peeled and sliced

In a large frying pan over a medium heat, cook the bacon until cooked through. Remove and set aside. Break the eggs into the pan, keeping them separate. Break the yolks open and cook until firm. Optionally, use a circular egg mould to maintain a 'clean' egg shape.

Spread 2 of the bread slices with 1 tablespoon of the mayo. Layer each with the reserved bacon, 1 egg and the avocado. Spread the remaining mayonnaise on top, and then top with the remaining 2 bread slices.

PER SERVING: 722 calories, 27g protein, 19g carbohydrates, 63g total fat, 14g saturated fat, 12g fibre, 855mg sodium

TEX-MEX EGG SALAD WRAPS

PREP TIME: 5 MINUTES | **TOTAL TIME:** 5 MINUTES

Makes 4 servings

Taco seasoning and Dijon mustard liven up old-fashioned egg salad to make a delicious wrap. Serve with one of the cream soups in this cookbook, such as Cream of Mushroom Soup with Chives (page 92), and you will be filled to bursting!

6 hard-boiled eggs, peeled and chopped

125g (4½oz) Mayonnaise (page 40 or shop-bought)

1 tbsp Dijon mustard or 2 tsp mustard powder

2 tsp Taco Seasoning Mix (page 57)

1 small onion, finely chopped

1 small tomato, finely chopped

4 Flaxseed Wraps (page 26)

90g (3oz) lettuce, salad leaves, baby spinach or rocket

In a large bowl, combine the eggs, mayonnaise, mustard, seasoning mix, onion and tomato. Mix thoroughly.

Place the wraps on a work surface. Divide the egg salad among the wraps, spreading it down the centre of each wrap. Top with the salad leaves. Roll up.

PER SERVING: 580 calories, 23g protein, 16g carbohydrates, 50g total fat, 12g saturated fat, 9g fibre, 460mg sodium

HOT CAPRESE SANDWICHES

PREP TIME: 5 MINUTES | **TOTAL TIME:** 5 MINUTES

Makes 2 servings

If you love a simple but elegant Caprese salad, you'll love this equally simple and elegant sandwich based on the same theme!

Use ripe, juicy tomatoes, preferably beefsteak or any vine-ripened varieties you can find (or grow!).

4 slices Basic Focaccia (page 21)

50g (2oz) sliced mozzarella cheese

2 medium tomatoes, sliced

12 medium to large fresh basil leaves, sliced lengthwise

3–4 tsp Spicy Italian Dressing (page 49)

Place 1 slice of focaccia on a plate and layer with the cheese and tomatoes. Scatter the basil over each. Drizzle with the dressing. Top with another slice of bread.

One at a time, microwave on high power for 30 to 60 seconds to melt the cheese. Or heat in a 160°C/325°F/Gas mark 3 oven for 3 to 4 minutes, or until the cheese is melted.

PER SERVING: 728 calories, 30g protein, 26g carbohydrates, 60g total fat, 10g saturated fat, 14g fibre, 1,031mg sodium

BALSAMIC MUSHROOM WRAPS

PREP TIME: 5 MINUTES | **TOTAL TIME:** 15 MINUTES

Makes 4 servings

Mushrooms – which are rich in potassium, niacin, trace minerals, soluble fibre and unique phytochemicals – are unsung heroes of nutrition, so you can never get too much of them! They are increasingly being recognized as providing unique anti-inflammatory, immune-enhancing, even cancer-protective effects.

Another variation on this basic theme: use large mushrooms, slice them and grill. Add the grilled mushroom slices to the wraps before rolling.

2 tbsp olive oil

1 small onion, finely chopped

450g (1lb) sliced portobello or button mushrooms

1 medium green pepper, sliced

1 garlic clove, finely chopped

2 tbsp balsamic vinegar

½ tsp sea salt

4 Flaxseed Wraps (page 26)

90g (3oz) baby spinach, rocket or lettuce

In a large frying pan over a medium heat, heat the oil. Cook the onion, mushrooms and pepper for 2 minutes, stirring frequently. Add the garlic and cook for 1 minute. Add the vinegar and salt. Cook for 3 minutes, or until the vinegar has nearly evaporated.

Place the wraps on a work surface. Spread the mushroom mixture down the centre of each wrap. Top with the salad leaves. Roll up.

PER SERVING: 345 calories, 16g protein, 19g carbohydrates, 26g total fat, 7g saturated fat, 11g fibre, 450mg sodium

PEPPERONI PIZZA WRAPS

PREP TIME: 5 MINUTES | **TOTAL TIME:** 10 MINUTES

Makes 4 servings

This wrap is almost *too* quick and easy! As with many dishes in our world minus wheat, don't let the modest size fool you: These simple wraps are deceptively filling. As with conventional pizza, this basic recipe can be easily modified: add sautéed onions and green peppers; replace the pepperoni with salami, sausage or minced beef; add provolone, Parmesan or goat's cheese.

4 Flaxseed Wraps (page 26)

125g (4½ oz) pizza sauce or tomato sauce

50g (2oz) pepperoni, sliced

225g (8oz) mozzarella cheese, grated or sliced

Place each wrap on a plate. Spread the pizza sauce or tomato sauce down the centre of each wrap. Top with the pepperoni and sprinkle with cheese.

One at a time, microwave on high power for 30 to 60 seconds or grill for 30 to 60 seconds under the grill to melt the cheese. Roll up.

PER SERVING: 553 calories, 28g protein, 14g carbohydrates, 44g total fat, 22g saturated fat, 7g fibre, 1,178mg sodium

SMOKED SALMON WRAPS

PREP TIME: 5 MINUTES | **TOTAL TIME:** 5 MINUTES

Makes 4 servings

Smoked salmon and cream cheese are a simple dietary pleasure, but, of course, the bagels for this treat are forbidden in our wheat-free lifestyle. So here's a replacement version of the familiar smoked salmon and bagels that uses wheat-free tortillas but keeps the comforting flavours of cream cheese, salmon and chives.

4 Tortillas (page 29)

110g (4oz) cream cheese, at room temperature

110g (4oz) smoked salmon

2 tbsp capers, drained

2 tbsp finely chopped fresh chives

Place the tortillas on a work surface. Spread the cream cheese in a thin layer over each tortilla. Top evenly with the salmon. Arrange the capers down the centre of each. Sprinkle the chives over each tortilla. Roll up.

PER SERVING: 293 calories, 16g protein, 10g carbohydrates, 24g total fat, 7g saturated fat, 8g fibre, 963mg sodium

TUNA–SPINACH BURGERS

PREP TIME: 15 MINUTES | **TOTAL TIME:** 25 MINUTES

Makes 4 servings

These healthy Tuna–Spinach Burgers, served as is or between two slices of Sandwich Bread (page 20) or Basic Focaccia (page 21), can be varied by simply choosing among the different seasoning mixes.

3 tbsp extra-virgin olive oil, divided

170g (6oz) fresh baby spinach

2 tins (150g/5oz each) wild-caught tuna, drained

½ small red pepper, finely chopped

1 tbsp Dijon mustard

2 tbsp Mayonnaise (page 40 or shop-bought)

1 tsp fish seasoning or seasoning mix of choice (pages 55–59)

1 egg

35g (1¼oz) Parmesan cheese, finely grated

25g (1oz) chickpea flour

In a large frying pan over a medium-high heat, heat 1 tablespoon of the oil until hot. Cook the spinach, stirring frequently, for 2 minutes, or just until wilted. Place in a mesh colander and press the excess liquid from the spinach. Coarsely chop.

In a medium bowl, with a fork or the back of a spoon, break the tuna up into small pieces. Add the chopped spinach, pepper, mustard, mayonnaise, seasoning mix and egg. Mix together until well combined. Stir in the cheese and chickpea flour and mix well. Shape the mixture into 4 burgers, about 9cm (3½in) in diameter.

In the same pan over a medium heat, heat the remaining 2 tablespoons oil until hot. Cook the burgers for 6 minutes, turning once, or until golden brown and heated through.

PER SERVING: 365 calories, 27g protein, 10g carbohydrates, 24g total fat, 4g saturated fat, 3g fibre, 798mg sodium

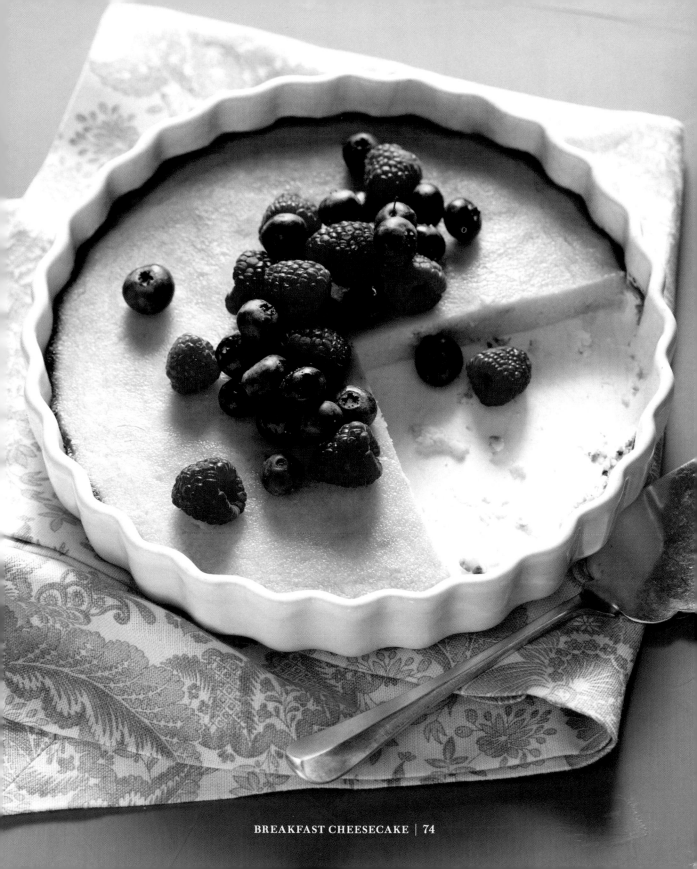

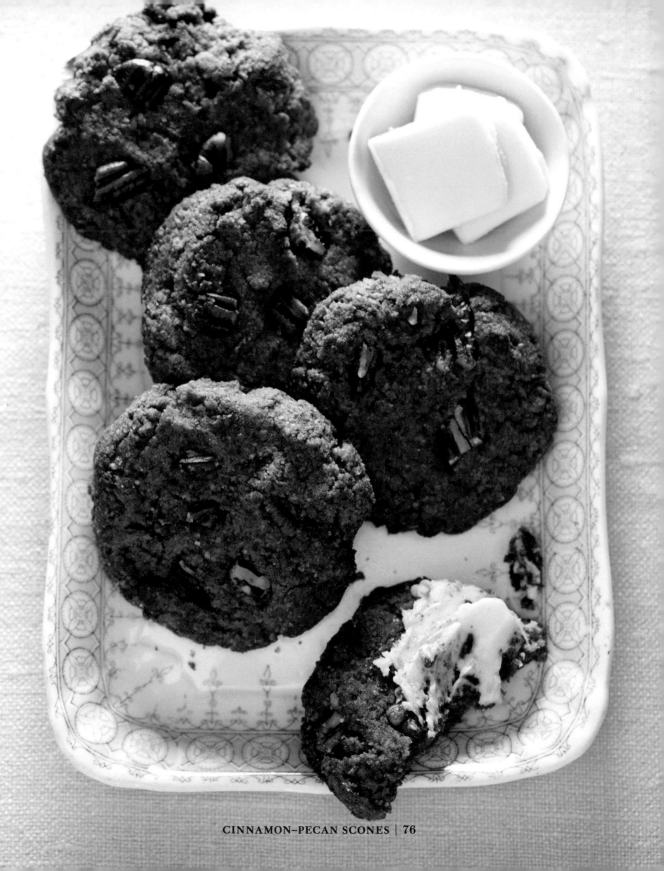

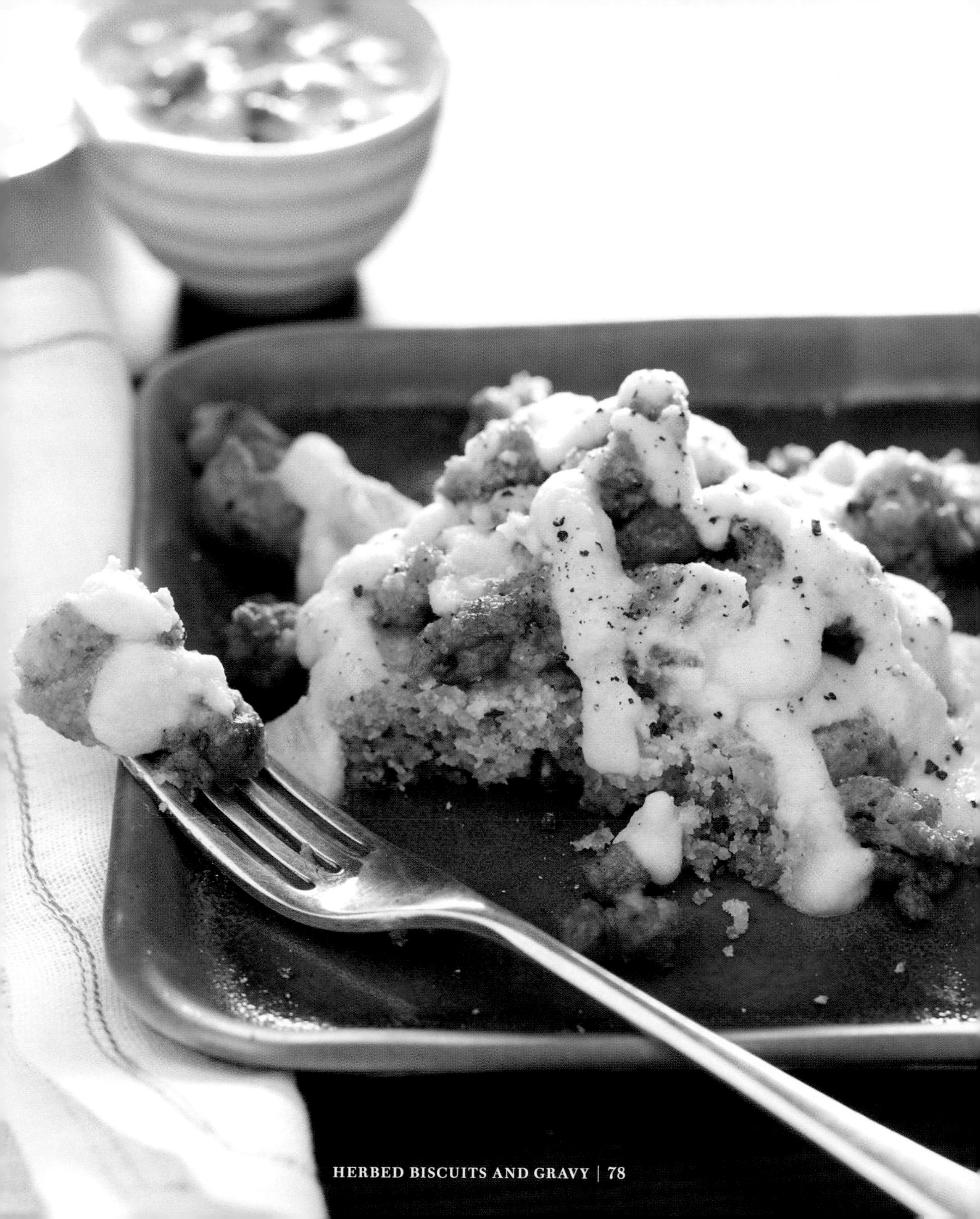

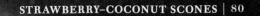

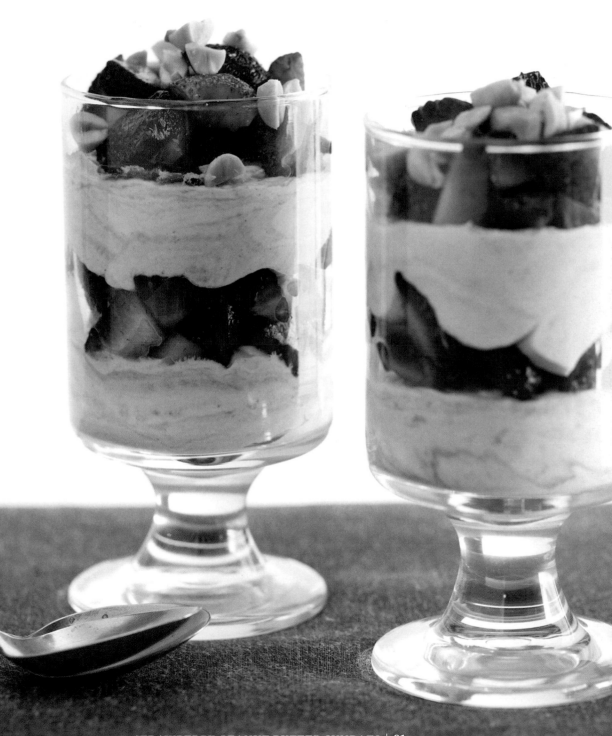

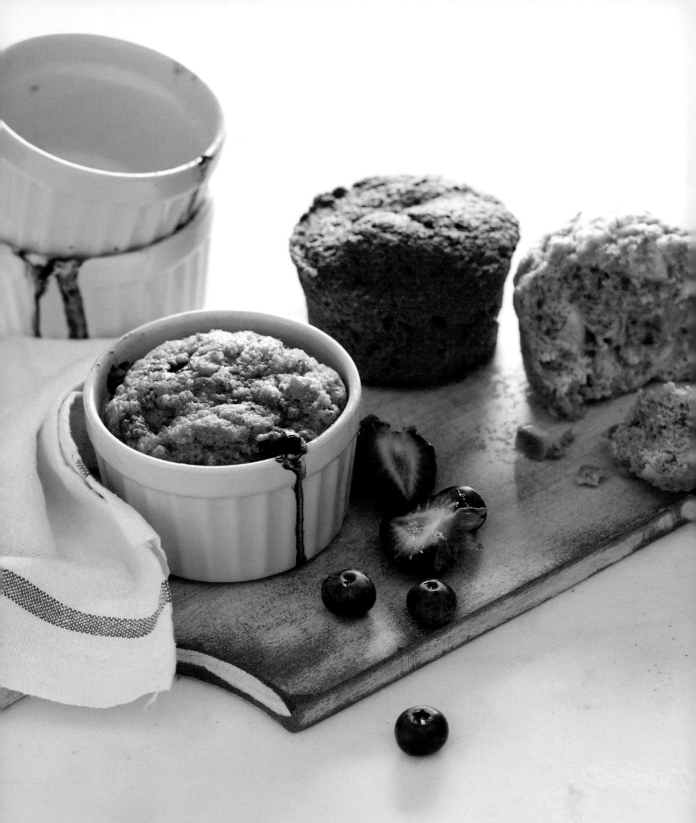

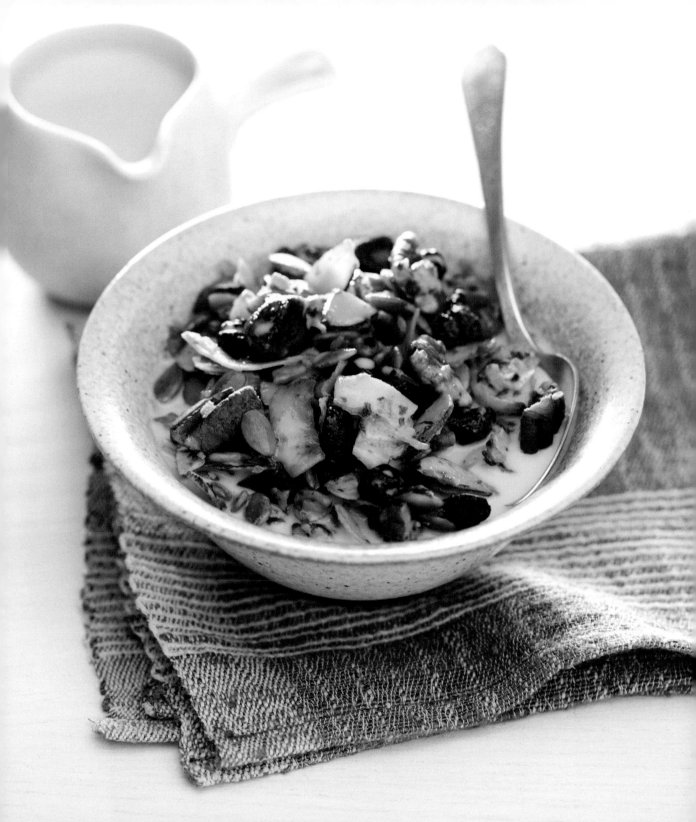

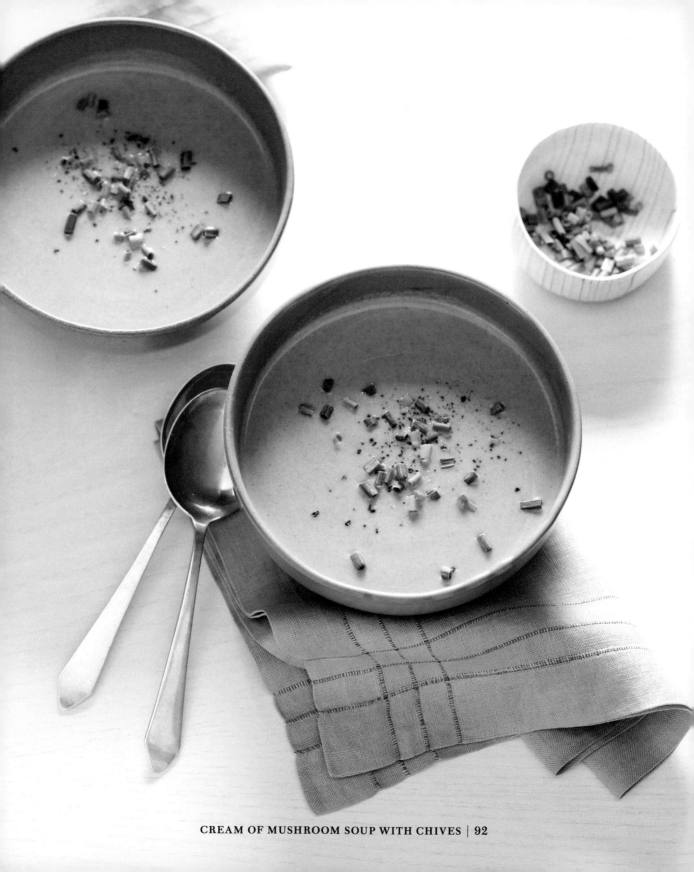

CREAM OF MUSHROOM SOUP WITH CHIVES | 92

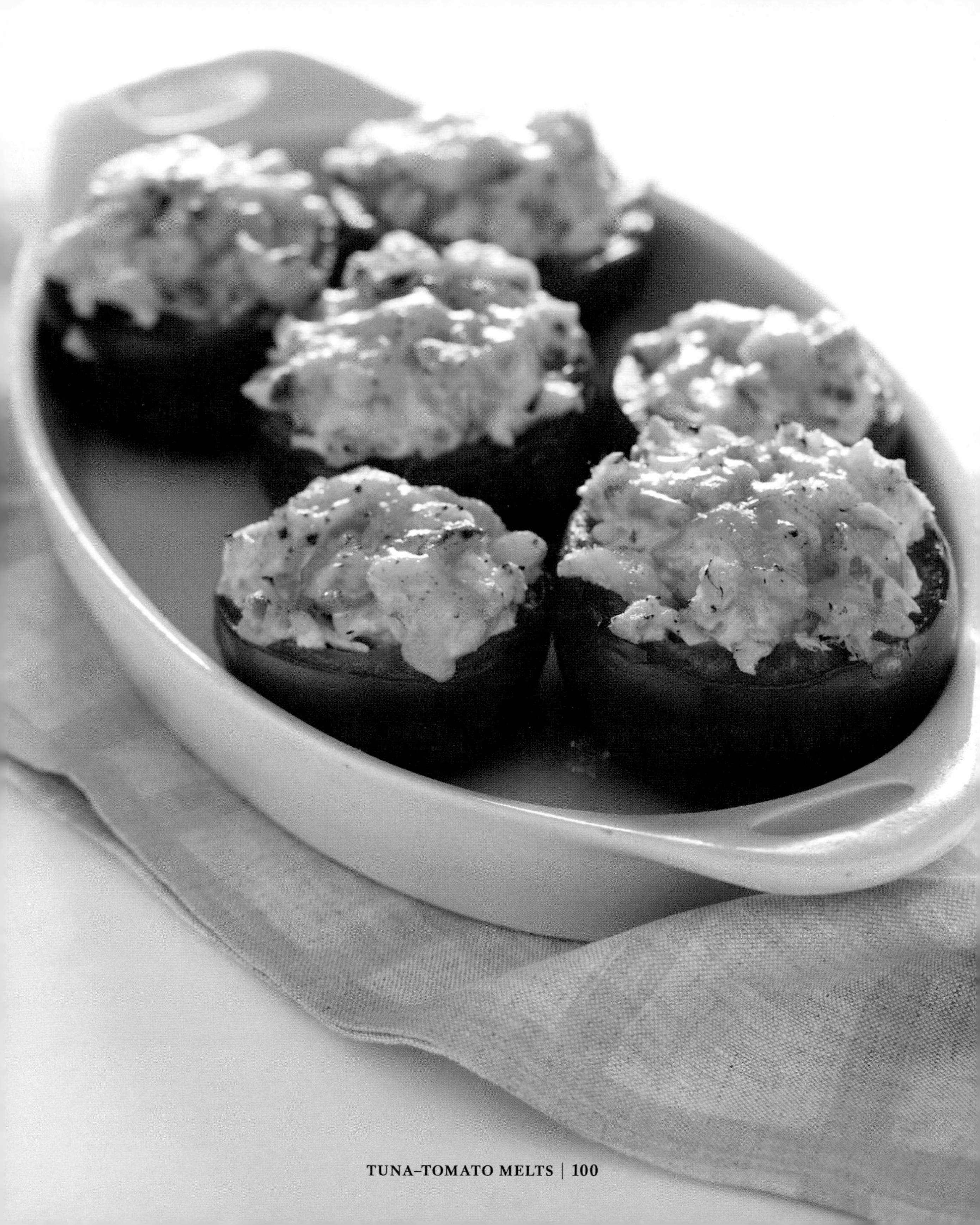

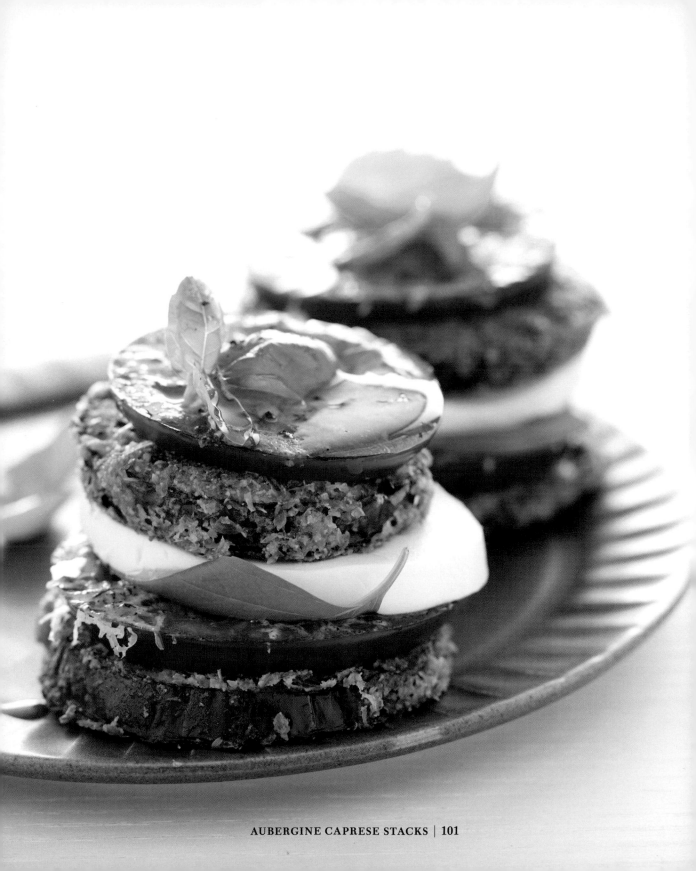

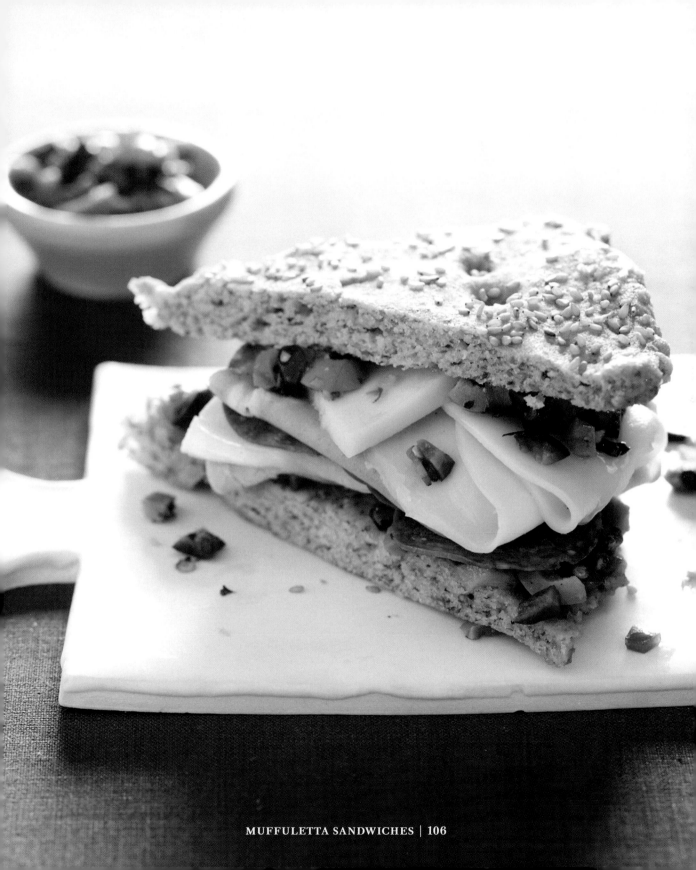

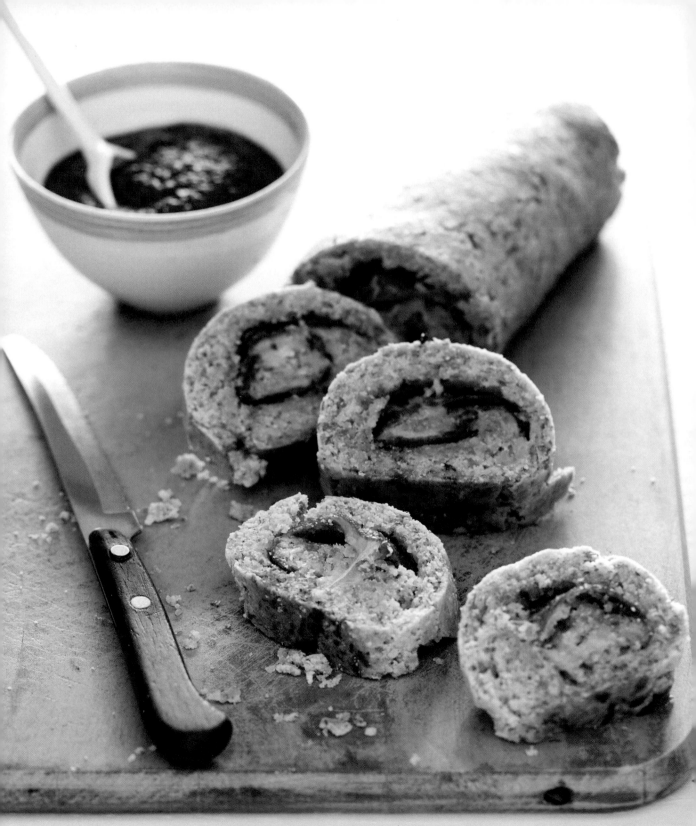

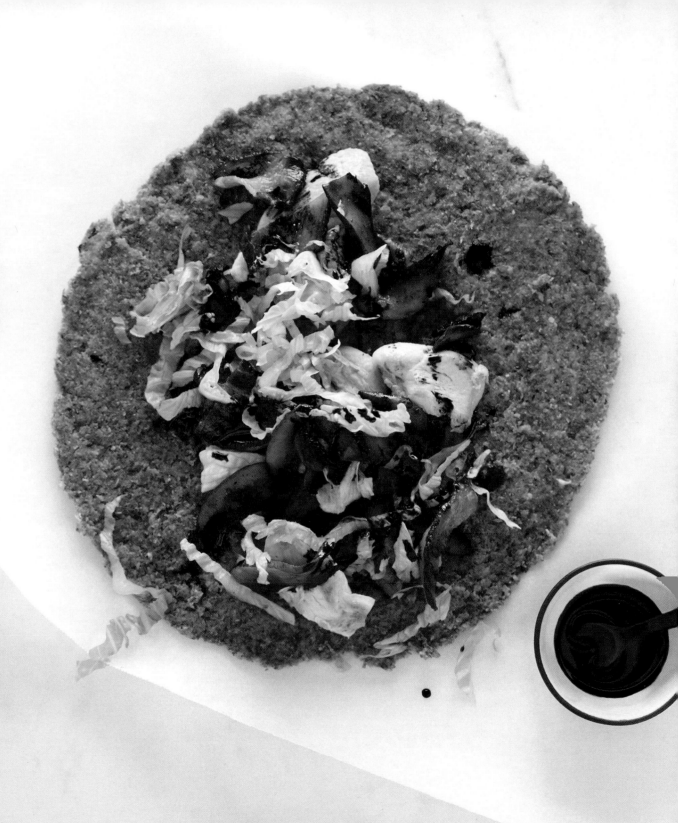

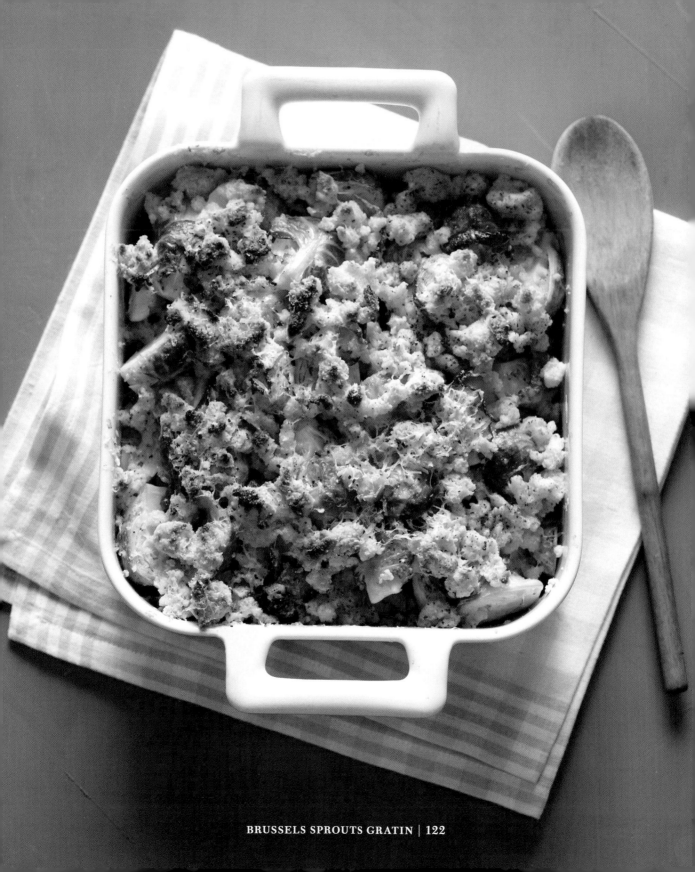

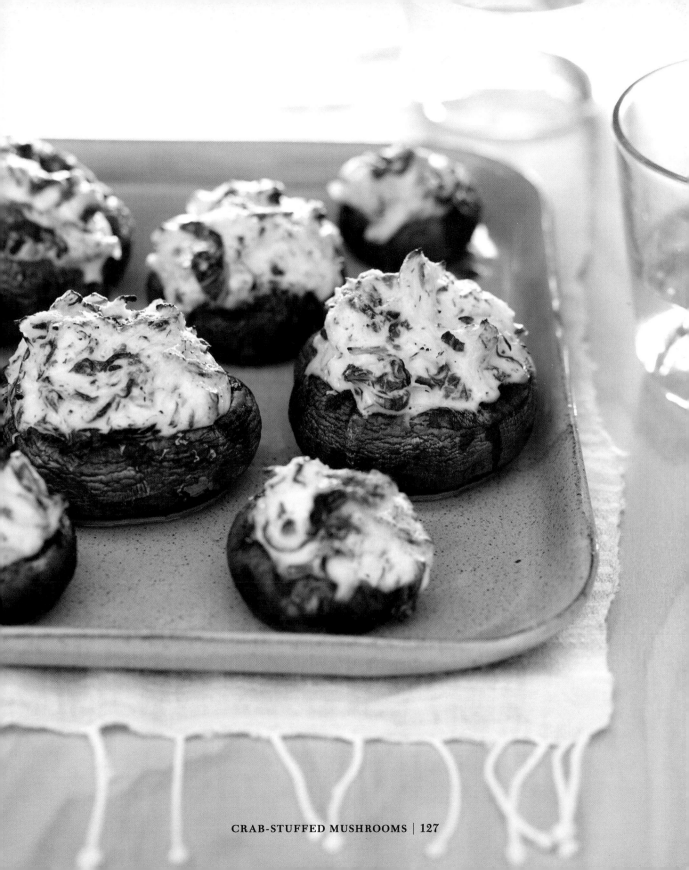

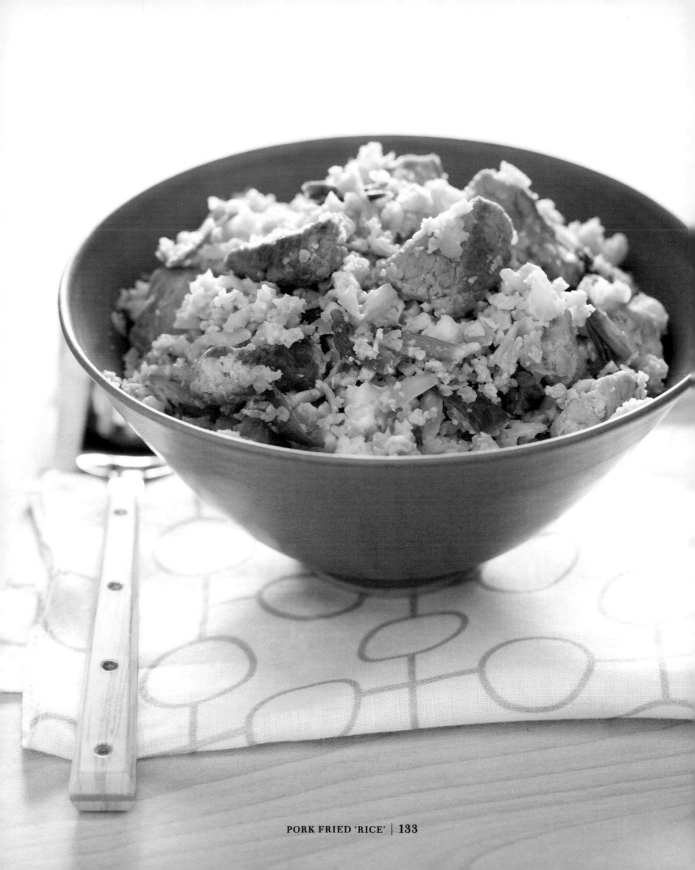

COURGETTE CAKES

PREP TIME: 10 MINUTES | **TOTAL TIME:** 20 MINUTES

Makes 4 servings

There are a number of different ways to enjoy these Italian-seasoned Courgette Cakes. I like serving them topped with Tomato Sauce (page 34) as a side dish for dinner or topped with a fried or poached egg for breakfast. They can also be broken up into pieces to make an interesting topping to a salad, replacing the croutons, served with Spicy Italian Dressing (page 49).

1 courgette, grated

1 egg, slightly beaten

2 tsp Italian Seasoning Mix (page 56)

75g (3oz) grated mozzarella cheese

25g (1oz) Parmesan cheese, grated

30g (1¼oz) ground golden flaxseeds

2 tbsp olive oil

Place the courgette in the centre of a clean piece of kitchen paper and wring or press out any excess moisture.

In a medium bowl, combine the courgette, egg, seasoning mix and mozzarella. Add the Parmesan and flaxseeds and stir to combine thoroughly. Divide the batter into 4 equal portions and form into 4 cakes, 1cm (½in) thick.

In a large frying pan over a medium-high heat, heat the oil until hot. Cook the cakes for 7 minutes, turning once, or until both sides are golden brown. Transfer to a plate lined with kitchen paper. Serve immediately.

PER SERVING: 192 calories, 10g protein, 5g carbohydrates, 16g total fat, 4g saturated fat, 3g fibre, 235mg sodium

ALMOND BUTTER AND JAM SANDWICH

PREP TIME: 5 MINUTES | **TOTAL TIME:** 5 MINUTES

Makes 1 serving

This is a more sophisticated adult version of the old PB & J sandwich! Almond butter replaces the peanut butter, but you can also use hazelnut butter, sunflower seed butter or whatever other nut or seed butter strikes your fancy. Likewise, you can alter the basic recipe provided for Plum–Chia Jam to use your choice of fruit.

2 slices Sandwich Bread (page 20)

1–2 tbsp almond butter

1 tbsp Plum–Chia Jam (page 51) or other no-sugar-added jams

On 1 slice of bread, spread the almond butter. Top with the jam and the remaining slice of bread.

PER SERVING: 456 calories, 17g protein, 18g carbohydrates, 39g total fat, 8g saturated fat, 9g fibre, 499mg sodium

ARTICHOKES, PANCETTA AND KALE WITH SHAVED PARMESAN

PREP TIME: 5 MINUTES | **TOTAL TIME:** 15 MINUTES

Makes 6 servings

The taste contrasts of the pancetta, artichokes, kale and Parmesan cheese make this dish a delight for the palate. While it can ably serve as a side dish alongside a wheat-free pasta dish or any meat, it can also make a healthy and filling stand-alone breakfast or lunch. For breakfast, top with a fried or poached egg.

If you don't have any pre-made Italian Seasoning Mix on hand, simply substitute 1 tablespoon dried oregano and 1 teaspoon dried rosemary.

2 tbsp extra-virgin olive oil

110g (4oz) pancetta, sliced into 2–3cm (1in) pieces

1 onion, finely chopped

2 garlic cloves, finely chopped

1 tsp Italian Seasoning Mix (page 56)

225g (8oz) chopped frozen, thawed, kale

1 jar or tin (350–400g/12–14oz) quartered artichokes, drained

50g (2oz) Parmesan cheese, shaved

In a large frying pan over a medium-high heat, heat the oil. Cook the pancetta, onion, garlic and Italian seasoning mix for 5 minutes, or until the pancetta is cooked through. If desired, drain off any excess oil.

Stir in the kale and artichokes. Reduce the heat to medium, cover, and cook for 5 minutes, or until the kale is wilted. Top with the cheese.

PER SERVING: 232 calories, 14g protein, 13g carbohydrates, 15g total fat, 4g saturated fat, 2g fibre, 1,336mg sodium

BRUSSELS SPROUTS GRATIN

PREP TIME: 5 MINUTES | **TOTAL TIME:** 30 MINUTES

Makes 4 servings

If you are new to the versatility of Brussels sprouts, let this dish get you acquainted! This is just one of the many ways to enjoy them – this time in a gratin dish.

As with all 30-minute meal dishes, don't let the butter and cheese fool you: minus wheat and other unhealthy ingredients, this dish easily fits into a slimming and healthy lifestyle.

I like serving this with lighter proteins, such as white fish or chicken.

450g (1lb) fresh Brussels sprouts, halved

225ml (8fl oz) water

3 tbsp butter, divided

25g (1oz) ground almonds/flour

40g (1½oz) Parmesan cheese, grated

¼ tsp sea salt

¼ tsp freshly ground black pepper

110ml (4fl oz) double cream

Preheat the oven to 200°C/400°F/Gas mark 6. Lightly grease a 2 litre (2 quart) baking dish.

In a microwaveable bowl, place the Brussels sprouts and water. Cover and microwave on high power for 5 minutes. Drain well and toss the Brussels sprouts with 1 tablespoon of the butter.

Meanwhile, in a small bowl, combine the ground almonds/flour, 25g (1oz) of the cheese, the salt and pepper. Using a pastry blender or 2 forks, cut the remaining 2 tablespoons butter into the flour mixture until crumbly.

Arrange the Brussels sprouts in the bottom of the baking dish. Pour the cream over the Brussels sprouts and sprinkle evenly with the crumb topping. Scatter the remaining 3 tablespoons cheese over the crumb topping.

Bake for 20 minutes, or until golden brown and bubbling.

PER SERVING: 310 calories, 10g protein, 13g carbohydrates, 26g total fat, 14g saturated fat, 5g fibre, 365mg sodium

BUTTERED CABBAGE

PREP TIME: 5 MINUTES | **TOTAL TIME:** 10 MINUTES

Makes 4 servings

Although ultra-simple, I include this Buttered Cabbage recipe because it both comfortably accompanies many of the main dishes in this cookbook and can also serve as the basis for a variety of interesting side dishes. For instance, start with bacon, pancetta or sausage before adding the cabbage; add Moroccan or Italian Seasoning Mix (pages 55 and 56) along with the salt and pepper; or replace the water with beef or chicken stock.

1 tbsp extra-virgin olive oil

450g (1lb) shredded cabbage or coleslaw mix

2 tbsp water

2 tbsp butter

¼ tsp sea salt

¼ tsp freshly ground black pepper

In a medium frying pan or wok over a medium-high heat, heat the oil until hot. Cook the cabbage, stirring constantly, for 3 minutes, or until it begins to soften. Add the water and continue to cook, stirring frequently, for 2 minutes, or until the cabbage is tender-crisp (or desired tenderness) and the water has evaporated. Add the butter and toss to coat. Season with the salt and pepper.

PER SERVING: 111 calories, 2g protein, 7g carbohydrates, 9g total fat, 4g saturated fat, 3g fibre, 170mg sodium

CAJUN KALE

PREP TIME: 5 MINUTES | **TOTAL TIME:** 30 MINUTES

Makes 4 servings

Using andouille or another smoked sausage introduces the heady spices of Cajun cooking to the earthy greenness of kale. If you like a bit more tang, add an extra tablespoon of vinegar.

This simple recipe is also easily converted to Cajun Kale Soup by increasing the chicken stock to 450ml (16fl oz), leaving out the vinegar, and seasoning with sea salt to taste.

2 tbsp extra-virgin olive oil, divided

1 andouille or another smoked sausage link (75g/3oz), diced

1 garlic clove, finely chopped

450g (1lb) frozen kale, thawed

110ml (4fl oz) chicken stock

¼ tsp crushed red chillies (optional)

1 tbsp apple cider vinegar

In a medium saucepan or wok over a medium heat, heat 1 tablespoon of the oil until hot. Cook the sausage for 4 minutes, or until lightly browned. Add the garlic and cook for 1 minute, stirring frequently. Transfer to a small plate and set aside.

In the same saucepan or wok, heat the remaining 1 tablespoon oil. Cook the kale, stirring constantly, for 2 minutes, or until coated with the oil and sizzling. Add the stock, cover, and cook, stirring occasionally, for 10 minutes, or until the kale is tender. Uncover and stir in the pepper flakes (if desired), vinegar, the reserved sausage and garlic and the collected juices. Cook for 5 minutes, or until the liquid has nearly evaporated.

PER SERVING: 143 calories, 7g protein, 7g carbohydrates, 11g total fat, 2g saturated fat, 2g fibre, 225mg sodium

HERBES DE PROVENCE MUSHROOMS

PREP TIME: 5 MINUTES | **TOTAL TIME:** 15 MINUTES

Makes 4 servings

These ultra-simple spicy mushrooms burst with the flavours of the Herbes de Provence. They make an interesting and healthy accompaniment to steak or pork. They also make a tasty addition to a Mediterranean salad.

225g (8oz) chestnut or baby portobello mushrooms

2 tbsp extra-virgin olive oil

1 tsp Herbes de Provence (page 59)

Preheat the oven to 180°C/350°F/Gas mark 4.

In a medium bowl, toss the mushrooms with the oil. Sprinkle with the Herbes de Provence and stir to coat evenly.

Place the mushrooms on a baking sheet. Bake for 10 minutes, tossing twice, or until browned.

PER SERVING: 77 calories, 1g protein, 3g carbohydrates, 7g total fat, 1g saturated fat, 1g fibre, 4mg sodium

ITALIAN MARINATED MUSHROOMS

PREP TIME: 5 MINUTES | **TOTAL TIME:** 20 MINUTES

Makes 4 servings

Super-duper quick and easy, these marinated mushrooms can be served as a starter or a side dish with steak, salmon or baked chicken. Quick variations can be made by adding one or more finely chopped fresh herbs, such as oregano or marjoram.

2 tbsp extra-virgin olive oil

450g (1lb) button or field mushrooms, stems removed

115ml (4fl oz) Spicy Italian Dressing (page 49)

In a large frying pan over a medium heat, heat the oil. Cook the mushrooms, stirring occasionally, covered, for 10 minutes, or until softened. Add the dressing and simmer for 3 minutes, or until the dressing is reduced by half.

PER SERVING: 260 calories, 3g protein, 5g carbohydrates, 26g total fat, 4g saturated fat, 1g fibre, 105mg sodium

CRAB-STUFFED MUSHROOMS

PREP TIME: 15 MINUTES | **TOTAL TIME:** 30 MINUTES

Makes 6 servings

Crab plus cream cheese plus mushrooms make a delicious, healthy and surprisingly filling starter. I replace the usual breadcrumbs with grated Parmesan cheese for a bit of crunch that also browns nicely in the oven.

275g (10oz) frozen chopped spinach, thawed and squeezed dry

1 tin (170g/6oz) crabmeat, drained

225g (8oz) cream cheese, softened

1 shallot, finely chopped

½ tsp dried dill

½ tsp sea salt

2 tbsp grated Parmesan cheese, divided

12 mushrooms, approximately 8–10cm (3–4in) diameter

Preheat the oven to 200°C/400°F/Gas mark 6.

In a medium bowl, combine the spinach, crabmeat, cream cheese, shallot, dill, salt and 1 tablespoon of the cheese.

Remove and discard the mushroom stems. Spoon the crab mixture into the stem side of the mushrooms and arrange on a baking sheet. Sprinkle the remaining 1 tablespoon cheese over the tops.

Bake for 15 minutes, or until the tops are golden and the mushrooms begin to release their juices.

PER SERVING: 227 calories, 12g protein, 12g carbohydrates, 14g total fat, 8g saturated fat, 3g fibre, 446mg sodium

SPINACH GRATIN

PREP TIME: 10 MINUTES | **TOTAL TIME:** 25 MINUTES

Makes 4 servings

This extra-cheesy spinach is a great way to get the kids (husbands included) to eat their spinach! Oozing with the smooth creaminess of a combination of double cream, cream cheese, butter and melted Parmesan cheese, this dish is sure to get requests for seconds!

1 tbsp extra-virgin olive oil

450g (1lb) fresh baby spinach

1 tbsp butter

2 tbsp cream cheese

6 tbsp double cream

50g (2oz) Parmesan cheese, grated, divided

¼ tsp sea salt

¼ tsp freshly ground black pepper

25g (1oz) ground almonds/flour

Place an oven rack in the middle of the oven and preheat the grill. Lightly grease a 1½ litre (1½ quart) baking dish.

In a large frying pan over a medium heat, heat the oil until hot. Cook the spinach, tossing occasionally with tongs, for 4 minutes, or just until wilted. Push the spinach towards the sides of the pan. Add the butter, cream cheese and cream to the centre of the pan and stir for 2 minutes, or until melted and hot. Add half of the Parmesan, the salt and pepper. Stir the spinach and sauce together. Pour into the baking dish.

In a small bowl, combine the ground almonds/flour and the remaining Parmesan. Sprinkle evenly over the spinach mixture.

Grill for 3 minutes, or until the topping is browned and the spinach is bubbly.

PER SERVING: 277 calories, 6g protein, 14g carbohydrates, 24g total fat, 11g saturated fat, 6g fibre, 338mg sodium

128 | LIGHT MEALS AND SIDE DISHES

ANGEL HAIR SQUASH

PREP TIME: 10 MINUTES | **TOTAL TIME:** 15 MINUTES

Makes 4 servings

The first time I heard someone suggest the use of squash as a noodle replacement, I was sceptical. But once you give it a try, you will be pleasantly surprised at how wonderfully this healthy substitute takes the place of wheat pasta (or other unhealthy replacements), with *none* of the adverse health potential.

5 small yellow squash

1 tbsp extra-virgin olive oil

1 tbsp butter

¼ tsp sea salt

Using a julienne vegetable slicer, mandolin or spiral slicer, cut the squash into matchsticks. In a large frying pan over a medium-high heat, heat the oil until hot. Cook the squash, stirring frequently, for 2–3 minutes, or just until it begins to wilt and softens slightly (do not overcook). Stir in the butter until melted and season with the salt.

PER SERVING: 96 calories, 3g protein, 8g carbohydrates, 7g total fat, 2g saturated fat, 3g fibre, 129mg sodium

COURGETTE NOODLES

PREP TIME: 5 MINUTES | **TOTAL TIME:** 10 MINUTES

Makes 4 servings

Courgette makes an excellent noodle replacement. It really helps to have one of the handy spiral slicers, such as a Spirelli or Spiralizer, or a julienne vegetable slicer, so converting courgettes into noodles is a snap. You can still do quite well by carefully cutting your courgettes with a sharp knife, veggie peeler or mandolin.

½ tsp sea salt   900g (2lb) courgettes

In a medium saucepan, bring 2 litres (2 quarts) of water and the salt to the boil. Meanwhile, using a vegetable peeler or mandolin, cut the courgettes into long, thin, wide ribbon strips. Add the ribbons to the water, reduce the heat to simmering and cook for 2 minutes, or until the courgette is soft and flexible. Drain in a colander and serve with your choice of sauce.

PER SERVING: 39 calories, 3g protein, 7g carbohydrates, 1g total fat, 0g saturated fat, 2g fibre, 94mg sodium

Note: This recipe can also be made in a frying pan. In a large non-stick pan over a medium-high heat, heat 2 tablespoons olive oil until hot. Cook the courgette ribbons, stirring frequently, for 3 to 4 minutes, or until al dente (do not overcook). Add 1 tablespoon butter and toss with the courgettes to melt. Season with salt to taste.

ROASTED COURGETTE, SQUASH AND TOMATO MEDLEY

PREP TIME: 10 MINUTES | **TOTAL TIME:** 30 MINUTES

Makes 4 servings

This colourful medley of vegetables is one of those recipes that can also serve as a vegetarian main meal or serve it with your choice of baked chicken, fish or pork.

1½ tbsp olive oil

1 tbsp red wine vinegar

½ tsp Italian Seasoning Mix (page 56)

½ tsp sea salt

2 small yellow squash, sliced into 5mm (¼in) thick half-moon slices

1 courgette, sliced into 5mm (¼in) thick half-moon slices

600g (1lb 5oz) cherry tomatoes, halved

35g (1¼oz) Parmesan cheese, finely shaved

Place an oven rack in the lower half of the oven and preheat the oven to 220°C/425°F/Gas mark 7.

In a large bowl, stir together the oil, vinegar, seasoning mix and salt. Add the squash, courgette and tomatoes and toss to coat. Spread the vegetables in a single layer on a large baking sheet.

Bake for 20 minutes, stirring once, or until the vegetables are browned. Sprinkle with the cheese.

PER SERVING: 129 calories, 5g protein, 11g carbohydrates, 8g total fat, 2g saturated fat, 2g fibre, 337mg sodium

CURRIED 'RICE'

PREP TIME: 5 MINUTES | **TOTAL TIME:** 15 MINUTES

Makes 4 servings

If you like the flavour of curry, you will love this simple Curried 'Rice' that uses the ever-versatile cauliflower as a grain-free replacement. For added spiciness, add a teaspoon of the Moroccan Seasoning Mix (page 48).

1 small head cauliflower, broken into
    large pieces

2 tbsp extra-virgin olive oil

1 onion, finely chopped

1 garlic clove, finely chopped

1–2 tsp curry powder

½ tsp sea salt

Using a food processor with a shredding disc attachment or the largest holes of a box grater, grate the cauliflower. Place in a microwaveable bowl. Cover and microwave on high power for 4 minutes, stirring once, or until it reaches the desired doneness.

Meanwhile, in a large frying pan over a medium heat, heat the oil. Cook the onion for 3 minutes, or until it begins to soften. Add the garlic and curry powder and cook for 1 minute, or until the curry is incorporated.

Add the steamed cauliflower and salt and stir to combine and heat through.

PER SERVING: 93 calories, 2g protein, 6g carbohydrates, 7g total fat, 1g saturated fat, 2g fibre, 218mg sodium

PORK FRIED 'RICE'

PREP TIME: 10 MINUTES | **TOTAL TIME:** 20 MINUTES

Makes 6 servings

Don't you love the pork fried rice you get at your local Chinese restaurant? Here it is, re-created with healthy ingredients but without MSG, wheat, cornflour or rice.

Chicken, beef and prawns or other shellfish can readily serve as substitutes for the pork.

1 head cauliflower, broken into large
   pieces

2 tbsp coconut oil, divided

4 spring onions, sliced

2 garlic cloves, finely chopped

2 eggs, whisked

225g (8oz) pork fillet, cut into
   1cm (½in) cubes

50ml (2fl oz) tamari or gluten-free
   soy sauce

Using a food processor with a shredding disc attachment or the largest holes of a box grater, grate the cauliflower. Place in a microwaveable bowl. Cover and microwave on high power for 4 minutes, stirring once, or until it reaches the desired doneness.

Meanwhile, in a wok or large frying pan over a medium-high heat, heat 1 tablespoon of the oil until hot. Cook the spring onions and garlic for 2 minutes. Add the eggs and stir continuously until cooked through and lightly browned. Remove the egg mixture to a bowl and set aside.

Reduce the heat to medium. Add the remaining 1 tablespoon oil to the wok or pan. Cook the pork, stirring frequently, for 5 minutes, or until no longer pink. Stir in the tamari or soy sauce, steamed cauliflower and the reserved egg mixture. Cook, stirring, for 2 minutes, or until heated through.

PER SERVING: 141 calories, 13g protein, 6g carbohydrates, 7g total fat, 5g saturated fat, 2g fibre, 702mg sodium

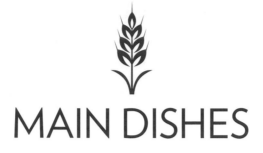

MAIN DISHES

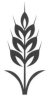

STEAK BÉARNAISE

PREP TIME: 5 MINUTES | **TOTAL TIME:** 15 MINUTES

Makes 4 servings

A French classic makes an appearance in the wheat-free lifestyle! Thick, rich and buttery béarnaise sauce transforms an ordinary steak into an event.

To save time, I've streamlined the classic method for making béarnaise – it's so simple, you can make it while the steaks are cooking.

4 fillet or sirloin steaks
   (170g/6oz each)

2 tbsp olive oil

¼ tsp sea salt

¼ tsp freshly ground black pepper

1 tbsp lemon juice

2 tsp white wine vinegar

1 shallot, finely chopped

2 egg yolks

2 tbsp chopped fresh tarragon, divided

110g (4oz) butter, melted

Pat both sides of the steaks dry using kitchen paper. Brush both sides with the oil and season with the salt and pepper.

Heat a well-seasoned indoor grill pan over a medium-high heat until hot. Cook the steaks for 6 minutes, turning once, or until a thermometer inserted in the centre registers 65°C (145°F) for medium-rare. Transfer the steaks to a platter.

Meanwhile, in a blender, combine the lemon juice, vinegar, shallot, egg yolks and 1 tablespoon of the tarragon. Blend for 30 seconds, or until creamy. With the blender running, pour the melted butter in a slow, steady stream into the yolk mixture, then continue to blend for 30 seconds. Remove to a serving vessel and stir in the remaining 1 tablespoon tarragon.

Top the steaks with the béarnaise sauce or serve on the side.

PER SERVING: 567 calories, 40g protein, 1g carbohydrates, 44g total fat, 21g saturated fat, 0g fibre, 403mg sodium

GINGER–SESAME PEPPER STEAK

PREP TIME: 15 MINUTES | **TOTAL TIME:** 25 MINUTES

Makes 4 servings

This simple stir-fried steak combined with the Asian flavours of ginger and sesame can make a substantial stand-alone main dish or can be served on top of shirataki noodles or 'riced' cauliflower.

450g (1lb) thin-sliced sirloin steak (about 1cm/½in thick)

2 tbsp coconut oil, divided

1 green pepper, cut into 5mm (¼in) strips

1 red or yellow pepper, cut into 5mm (¼in) strips

1 sweet onion, thinly sliced lengthwise

2 garlic cloves, finely chopped

1 tbsp grated fresh ginger

2 tbsp tamari or gluten-free soy sauce

2 tsp sesame oil

Slice the steak crosswise against the grain into 5mm (¼in) wide strips.

In a wok or large frying pan over a high heat, heat 1 tablespoon of the coconut oil until hot. Stir-fry the peppers and onion for 3 minutes, or until tender but still crisp. Transfer to a plate and set aside.

In the same wok or pan, heat the remaining 1 tablespoon coconut oil until hot. Cook the steak strips for 1 minute, stirring constantly. Add the garlic and ginger and stir-fry for 2 minutes, or until the steak is browned. Stir in the tamari or soy sauce and sesame oil. Return the reserved peppers and onion to the wok and cook for 1 minute, tossing, or until hot.

PER SERVING: 270 calories, 27g protein, 7g carbohydrates, 15g total fat, 8g saturated fat, 2g fibre, 540mg sodium

BEEF STROGANOFF

PREP TIME: 10 MINUTES | **TOTAL TIME:** 30 MINUTES

Makes 4 servings

Sure, beef Stroganoff is an old 20th-century favourite, but here I resurrect it minus all the unhealthy ingredients, creating a wonderful traditional dish for special occasions or a rich evening meal.

3 tbsp butter, divided

450g (1lb) sirloin or fillet beef, thinly sliced into 5mm (½in) strips

350g (12oz) sliced mushrooms (button or portobello)

3 shallots or 1 large onion, sliced

2 garlic cloves, finely chopped

110ml (4fl oz) beef stock

¼ tsp sea salt

¼ tsp freshly ground black pepper

225ml (8fl oz) soured cream

1 tbsp Dijon mustard

In a large frying pan over a medium-high heat, melt 1 tablespoon of the butter. Sear the beef for 2 minutes, turning once, or until browned on both sides and just barely cooked through. (Work in batches, if necessary.) Remove the beef to a plate and set aside. Return the pan to medium heat.

Add the remaining 2 tablespoons butter, the mushrooms, shallots or onion and garlic. Cook for 5 minutes, or until the shallots or onion is softened and the mushrooms release their juices. Stir in the reserved beef, the stock, salt and pepper. Bring to the boil, reduce the heat to medium-low, cover and simmer for 10 minutes.

Stir in the soured cream and mustard. Cook for 1 minute, or until heated through.

PER SERVING: 353 calories, 29g protein, 6g carbohydrates, 24g total fat, 13g saturated fat, 1g fibre, 406mg sodium

VEAL SCHNITZEL WITH LEMON WINE SAUCE

PREP TIME: 10 MINUTES | **TOTAL TIME:** 30 MINUTES

Makes 4 servings

Rediscover this traditional Austrian dish in our wheat-free world using almond flour and ground golden flaxseeds as the 'breading'. Optionally, serve with mashed cauliflower.

Some shops sell very thin veal escalopes. If you find thicker ones, pound them between 2 sheets of clingfilm with a meat mallet or frying pan to an even 5mm (¼in) thickness.

2 eggs

¾ tsp sea salt, divided

¾ tsp freshly ground black pepper, divided

55g (2oz) blanched almond flour

65g (2½oz) ground golden flaxseeds

½ tsp garlic powder

450g (1lb) veal escalopes, 2.5–5mm (⅛–¼in) thick

2 tbsp extra-virgin olive oil

50ml (2fl oz) dry white wine or chicken stock

2 tsp lemon juice

1 tbsp fresh parsley, finely chopped

2 tbsp butter, cubed and at room temperature

Preheat the oven to its lowest setting.

In a shallow bowl or pie tin or dish, lightly beat the eggs with ¼ teaspoon of the salt and ¼ teaspoon of the pepper.

In a separate shallow bowl or pie tin or dish, combine the flour, flaxseeds, garlic powder, the remaining ½ teaspoon salt, and the remaining ½ teaspoon pepper. Dip the veal escalopes into the egg, shaking off any excess. Dredge in the flour mixture. Place the breaded escalope on a plate. Repeat with the remaining escalopes.

In a large frying pan over a medium heat, heat the oil until hot. Cook the escalopes for 4 minutes, turning once, or until golden brown (add additional oil if necessary). Place the cooked escalopes on a baking sheet and keep warm in the oven.

Add the wine or stock and lemon juice to the pan, using a wooden spoon to loosen any browned bits on the bottom. Cook, stirring, for 2 minutes. Stir in the parsley. Remove the pan from the heat and whisk in the butter, 1 to 2 cubes at a time, until fully incorporated. Spoon the sauce over the escalopes.

PER SERVING: 387 calories, 32g protein, 7g carbohydrates, 26g total fat, 4g saturated fat, 6g fibre, 441mg sodium

BARBECUE BEEF QUESADILLAS

PREP TIME: 10 MINUTES | **TOTAL TIME:** 30 MINUTES

Makes 4 servings

The use of the Barbecue Sauce converts this dish, which is usually filled with sugar or high-fructose corn syrup, into something healthy but every bit as delicious as the original version. Serve as is, or with soured cream and guacamole.

2 tbsp extra-virgin olive oil, divided

110g (4oz) sirloin, bavette or rib-eye steak

½ tsp sea salt, divided

½ tsp freshly ground black pepper, divided

1 onion, quartered and thinly sliced

2 garlic cloves, finely chopped

1 green pepper, seeded and thinly sliced

100g (3½oz) Barbecue Sauce (page 35)

8 Tortillas (page 29)

125g (4½oz) Cheddar cheese, grated

In a large frying pan over a medium heat, heat 1 tablespoon of the oil until hot. Season the steak with ¼ teaspoon of the salt and ¼ teaspoon of the black pepper. Sear the steak for 5 minutes, turning once, or until browned on both sides. Remove from the frying pan and let rest for 5 minutes. Slice thinly.

Meanwhile, heat the remaining 1 tablespoon oil in the pan. Cook the onion, garlic, pepper, the remaining ¼ teaspoon salt and the remaining ¼ teaspoon black pepper for 5 minutes, stirring occasionally, or until the onion is translucent and the pepper softens. Remove from the heat, add the beef, and stir the barbecue sauce into the mixture.

Wipe the pan clean and heat over a medium heat. Place 1 tortilla in the centre. Sprinkle 1 tablespoon cheese on the tortilla and top with a quarter of the steak mixture. Sprinkle another tablespoon cheese over the steak mixture and set another tortilla on top. Cook for 2 minutes, turning once, or until both tortillas are golden and the cheese is melted. Remove and cover to keep warm. Repeat with the remaining tortillas and filling.

PER SERVING: 579 calories, 32g protein, 25g carbohydrates, 43g total fat, 10g saturated fat, 14g fibre, 845mg sodium

BEEF STEW

PREP TIME: 5 MINUTES | **TOTAL TIME:** 30 MINUTES

Makes 4 servings

Another old favourite makes a comeback sans wheat. This updated version adds some hearty vegetables along with a red wine sauce for added richness and health benefits.

450g (1lb) braising steak, cut into
2–3cm (1in) cubes

2 tbsp chickpea flour or coconut flour

2 tbsp extra-virgin olive oil

1 litre (1 quart) beef stock

450g (1lb) frozen vegetables (broccoli,
cauliflower and carrots)

2 tsp Italian Seasoning Mix (page 56)

1 tsp freshly ground black pepper

½ tsp sea salt

50ml (2fl oz) dry red wine

3 tbsp tomato purée

In a large resealable plastic bag, combine the cubed beef and flour. Shake well until the beef is coated.

In a large saucepan, heat the oil over a medium-high heat. Cook the beef, turning, for 10 minutes, or until browned on all sides.

Add the stock, vegetables, seasoning mix, pepper, salt and wine and bring to the boil. Reduce the heat to a simmer and cook for 10 minutes.

Add the tomato purée and cook for 5 minutes, or until thickened.

PER SERVING: 317 calories, 30g protein, 14g carbohydrates, 13g total fat, 3g saturated fat, 4g fibre, 502mg sodium

UNSTUFFED CABBAGE AND BEEF

PREP TIME: 5 MINUTES | **TOTAL TIME:** 30 MINUTES

Makes 4 servings

Don't let the simplicity of this healthy, wheat-free recipe fool you: it yields a delicious and filling final product that you will be proud to serve! If desired, this can be served over 'riced' cauliflower.

1 tbsp olive oil

450g (1lb) steak mince

1 small onion, chopped

1 tin (400g/14oz) chopped tomatoes

½ tsp sea salt

½ tsp freshly ground black pepper

450g (1lb) coleslaw or shredded cabbage mix

110ml (4fl oz) water

110ml (4fl oz) soured cream (optional)

In a large Dutch oven or frying pan with a lid over a medium-high heat, heat the oil. Cook the minced beef and onion, breaking the beef into small chunks, for 5 minutes, or until the beef is no longer pink and the onion is soft. Stir in the tomatoes, salt and pepper. Add the coleslaw or cabbage mix and water and stir until combined. Reduce the heat to medium, cover, and simmer, stirring occasionally, for 20 minutes, or until the cabbage is the desired doneness.

Remove from the heat and stir in the soured cream, if desired. Taste for seasoning and add more salt and pepper, if needed.

PER SERVING: 227 calories, 26g protein, 8g carbohydrates, 10g total fat, 2g saturated fat, 3g fibre, 374mg sodium

SLOPPY JOES

PREP TIME: 10 MINUTES | **TOTAL TIME:** 30 MINUTES

Makes 4 servings

This American favourite is simple to make and easily fits into a wheat-free lifestyle. Make the wheat-free bread (for example, Basic Sandwich Muffins, page 24) ahead of time to top with this Sloppy Joe mix as an open-faced sandwich.

If you make the rolls at the same time as the Sloppy Joe mix, allow an additional 10 minutes to make the rolls from the All-Purpose Baking Mix (page 19) so they can bake while the Sloppy Joe mixture is cooking on the hob.

450g (1lb) minced beef

1 small onion, chopped

1 green pepper, chopped

2 garlic cloves, finely chopped,
   or 1 tsp garlic powder

225g (8oz) tomato sauce

155g (5½oz) Barbecue Sauce (page 35)

½ tsp sea salt

In a large frying pan over a medium-high heat, cook the beef for 5 minutes, or until no longer pink. Add the onion, pepper and garlic or garlic powder and cook for 5 minutes, or until the vegetables soften. Drain. Reduce the heat to medium-low and stir in the tomato sauce, barbecue sauce and salt. Cover and cook for 10 minutes.

PER SERVING: 301 calories, 23g protein, 13g carbohydrates, 18g total fat, 7g saturated fat, 2g fibre, 728mg sodium

TACO LETTUCE WRAPS

PREP TIME: 5 MINUTES | **TOTAL TIME:** 15 MINUTES

Makes 4 servings

Make light but tasty Mexican wraps, spiced up with time-saving Taco Seasoning Mix, using a wheat-free lettuce wrap. Optionally, add some sliced onions and green peppers to the minced beef.

Top the wrap filling with chopped avocado, grateed Cheddar cheese, chopped tomatoes, soured cream or salsa.

570g (1¼lb) minced beef

1 tsp Taco Seasoning Mix
(page 57)

250g (9oz) tomato salsa

8 large leaves lettuce

Toppings: chopped avocado, grated
Cheddar cheese, chopped tomatoes,
soured cream, salsa

In a large frying pan over a medium-high heat, cook the beef and seasoning mix, breaking the beef up with a large spoon, for 5 minutes, or until no longer pink. Reduce the heat to medium, stir in the salsa and cook for 3 minutes, or until most of the liquid has evaporated.

To serve, divide the meat filling evenly among the lettuce. Top with the desired toppings. Roll up.

PER SERVING: 385 calories, 31g protein, 15g carbohydrates, 22g total fat, 8g saturated fat, 4g fibre, 450mg sodium

PEPPER AND BEEF TORTILLAS

PREP TIME: 10 MINUTES | **TOTAL TIME:** 20 MINUTES

Makes 4 servings

Now that you can make tortillas without wheat or corn, well, let's put them to good use! Here is one simple way to combine the Mexican flavours of the Taco Seasoning Mix with the fresh flavour of a sweet pepper, topped with cheese, of course!

Serve these tortillas with your favourite taco toppings, if desired: shredded lettuce, soured cream, chopped avocados or chopped fresh tomatoes.

2 tbsp extra-virgin olive oil

1 onion, finely chopped

1 poblano chilli or large sweet pepper, finely chopped (wear plastic gloves when handling)

2 garlic cloves, finely chopped

350g (12oz) minced beef

1 tbsp Taco Seasoning Mix (page 57)

½ tsp sea salt

1 large tomato, chopped

4 Tortillas (page 29)

125g (4½oz) Cheddar cheese, grated

In a large frying pan over a medium-high heat, heat the oil. Cook the onion, pepper and garlic for 3 minutes, or until softened. Add the beef, seasoning mix and salt and cook, stirring frequently, for 3 minutes, or until no longer pink.

Stir in the tomato, cover, and cook for 2 minutes, or until heated through. Spoon a quarter of the beef mixture over each tortilla. Sprinkle each with a quarter of the cheese and fold.

PER SERVING: 641 calories, 41g protein, 17g carbohydrates, 47g total fat, 17g saturated fat, 8g fibre, 881mg sodium

MIDDLE EASTERN LAMB BURGERS

PREP TIME: 10 MINUTES | **TOTAL TIME:** 20 MINUTES

Makes 4 servings

These unique burgers are rich with an exotic mix of flavours from mint and the Moroccan blend of seasonings. They combine especially well with the Dilled Cucumber Yoghurt Sauce (page 38).

450g (1lb) minced lamb

1 large garlic clove, finely chopped

1 small onion, grated

1 tsp dried mint

¾ tsp sea salt

1½ tsp Moroccan Seasoning Mix (page 48)

1 egg

2 tbsp extra-virgin olive oil

In a medium bowl, combine the lamb, garlic, onion, mint, salt, seasoning mix and egg until well combined. Divide the meat mixture into 4 burgers.

In a large frying pan over a medium heat, heat the oil until hot. Cook the patties for 8 minutes, turning once, or until browned and a thermometer inserted in the centre registers 70°C (160°F) for medium.

PER SERVING: 340 calories, 21g protein, 5g carbohydrates, 26g total fat, 12g saturated fat, 1g fibre, 394mg sodium

GRILLED PORK FILLET

PREP TIME: 5 MINUTES | **TOTAL TIME:** 20 MINUTES

Makes 4 servings

Enhanced with a seasoning mix (here I use the Cajun, but you can replace it with the Italian, Moroccan, Taco or your own mix of herbs and spices), a delicious grilled pork fillet requires just a few minutes of preparation and 15 or so minutes of grilling.

1 tbsp Cajun Seasoning Mix (page 58)

1 tsp sea salt

675g (1½lb) pork fillet

315g (11oz) Barbecue Sauce (page 35), divided

Grease the grill rack. If using an overhead grill, set the heat to medium-high. If using an oven grill, set the rack 15 to 20cm (6 to 8in) from the heat source and preheat to high.

In a small bowl, combine the seasoning mix and salt.

Slice the silver skin off the pork (but leave the fat, it's good for you!). Rub the seasoning mixture into the pork. Place half of the barbecue sauce in a small bowl and set aside.

Place the pork on the grill rack. Grill for 8 minutes, turning once. Brush with the remaining barbecue sauce. Grill for 7 minutes, turning once, or until a thermometer inserted in the centre reaches 70°C (160°F) and the juices run clear. Slice and serve with the reserved barbecue sauce.

PER SERVING: 222 calories, 36g protein, 8g carbohydrates, 4g total fat, 1g saturated fat, 1g fibre, 753mg sodium

DIJON MUSTARD PORK FILLET MEDALLIONS

PREP TIME: 5 MINUTES | **TOTAL TIME:** 25 MINUTES

Makes 4 servings

Pork fillet is a pretty classy dish to start with. But here's an even classier combination of Dijon mustard and white wine that your family and guests will think required hours to prepare. For greatest flavour, leave the fat on the fillet.

2 tbsp extra-virgin olive oil

675g (1½lb) pork fillet, cut into 1–2cm (½–¾in) thick slices

1 shallot, finely chopped

225g (8oz) mushrooms, thinly sliced

60g (2½oz) Dijon mustard

50ml (2fl oz) double cream or tinned coconut milk

2 tbsp white wine

½ tsp sea salt

In a large frying pan over a high heat, heat the oil. Working in batches if necessary, cook the pork slices for 4 minutes, turning once, or until browned. Transfer to a plate.

Reduce the heat to medium. Cook the shallot and mushrooms, stirring frequently, for 5 minutes, or until the mushrooms are softened. Stir in the mustard, cream or coconut milk, wine and salt. Cook for 4 minutes, stirring occasionally, or until blended. Return the pork medallions to the pan, cover, and cook for 5 minutes, or until the flavours blend and the pork is cooked through.

PER SERVING: 353 calories, 38g protein, 10g carbohydrates, 16g total fat, 6g saturated fat, 1g fibre, 657mg sodium

ITALIAN PORK FILLET

PREP TIME: 5 MINUTES | **TOTAL TIME:** 30 MINUTES

Makes 4 servings

Pork fillet is an easy, delicious cut of meat that eagerly takes on the flavours of herbs and spices that surround it. The combined herbs of the Italian Seasoning Mix are used in this dish. For the best flavour, don't trim the fat off the fillet.

This dish makes great leftovers for lunch or even breakfast.

2 tbsp extra-virgin olive oil

675g (1½lb) pork fillet

4 garlic cloves, finely chopped

1 tin (400g/14oz) quartered artichoke hearts, drained

60g (2½oz) roasted red peppers, sliced

1 onion, halved and sliced

2 tsp Italian Seasoning Mix (page 56)

In a large frying pan over a medium-high heat, heat the oil. Cook the pork, turning as necessary, for 15 minutes, or until a thermometer inserted in the centre reaches 70°C (160°F) and the juices run clear. Transfer to a serving plate and cover with foil to keep warm.

Reduce the heat to medium. Cook the garlic, artichokes, peppers, onion and seasoning mix, stirring occasionally, for 10 minutes, or until the onion is softened. Serve the vegetables with the pork.

PER SERVING: 310 calories, 38g protein, 14g carbohydrates, 11g total fat, 2g saturated fat, 3g fibre, 494mg sodium

SRIRACHA PORK AND AUBERGINE

PREP TIME: 15 MINUTES | **TOTAL TIME:** 30 MINUTES

Makes 4 servings

If you are a fan of hot pepper, you will love this extra-spicy pork and aubergine dish exploding with the unique flavours of Sriracha hot chilli sauce. But be warned: this is for the true lover of hot and spicy! Or, reduce the Sriracha to 1 tablespoon to still get the delicious flavours without all the fire.

3 tbsp extra-virgin olive oil or coconut oil, divided

675g (1½lb) pork fillet, cut into 2–3cm (1in) cubes

1 aubergine, cut into 1cm (½in) cubes

1 large onion, halved and thinly sliced

1 large green pepper, thinly sliced

2–4 tbsp Sriracha hot chilli sauce

110ml (4fl oz) water

In a large frying pan over a medium-high heat, heat 1 tablespoon of the oil. Cook the pork for 5 minutes, turning occasionally, or until browned. Remove to a plate. Add the remaining 2 tablespoons oil to the pan. Cook the aubergine, onion and pepper for 3 minutes, stirring constantly. Stir in the Sriracha sauce, water, pork and any accumulated juices. Reduce the heat to medium, cover, and cook for 10 minutes, stirring occasionally, or until the vegetables are softened and the pork is cooked through.

PER SERVING: 345 calories, 38g protein, 15g carbohydrates, 15g total fat, 3g saturated fat, 5g fibre, 247mg sodium

PORK MEDALLIONS WITH APPLE PAN SAUCE

PREP TIME: 15 MINUTES | **TOTAL TIME:** 25 MINUTES

Makes 4 servings

This pork dish is substantial enough to serve at celebrations or to make an extra-special evening meal. The reduced apple juice and apple cider vinegar, along with thyme and butter, provide a rich dimension to the meaty flavours of the pork fillet. Don't trim the fat off your fillet, by the way, for added flavour.

Optionally, serve this dish with Buttered Cabbage (page 123).

55g (2oz) ground almonds/flour

¼ tsp sea salt

¼ tsp dried thyme

675g (1½lb) pork fillet, cut into 5mm (¼in) slices

2 tbsp extra-virgin olive oil

2 tbsp butter, divided

1 shallot, finely chopped

225ml (8fl oz) apple juice (no sugar added)

2 tbsp apple cider vinegar

On a plate, combine the flour, salt and thyme. Dredge each pork medallion in the flour mixture to coat lightly and shake off excess.

In a large pan over a medium-high heat, heat the oil. Cook the pork for 3 minutes, turning once, or until golden brown. Transfer to a plate and loosely cover with foil to keep warm.

In the same pan, melt 1 tablespoon of the butter. Cook the shallot, stirring constantly, for 1 minute, or until it begins to soften. Add the apple juice and vinegar and cook for 2 minutes, stirring to loosen any brown bits on the bottom of the pan. Reduce the heat to medium-low and simmer for 5 minutes, or until the sauce has reduced by half. Stir in the remaining 1 tablespoon butter until melted.

Return the pork to the pan, along with any accumulated juices, and heat for 1 minute, or until heated through.

PER SERVING: 421 calories, 39g protein, 13g carbohydrates, 24g total fat, 6g saturated fat, 2g fibre, 247mg sodium

JAMBALAYA

PREP TIME: 15 MINUTES | **TOTAL TIME:** 30 MINUTES

Makes 4 servings

Treat your family to this little hint of New Orleans spicy Cajun-style cooking while devoting just a few minutes to the effort!

While there are many variations on the traditional Creole dish, this version is free of wheat and sugars. It can be served as is alongside a steamed vegetable, or on top of 'riced' cauliflower.

3 tbsp extra-virgin olive oil or coconut oil, divided

1 onion, finely chopped

2 garlic cloves, finely chopped

1 jalapeño or other green chilli, seeded and minced (wear plastic gloves when handling)

450g (1lb) andouille or smoked sausage, sliced

225g (8oz) chicken breast, cut into 2–3cm (1in) cubes

1–2 tbsp Cajun Seasoning Mix (page 58)

1 tin (400g/14oz) chopped tomatoes

170g (6oz) fresh baby spinach

In a large frying pan over a medium-high heat, heat 2 tablespoon of the oil until hot. Cook the onion, garlic and pepper for 3 minutes, or until they begin to soften.

Add the remaining 1 tablespoon oil to the pan. Stir in the sausage and chicken. Cover and cook for 5 minutes, stirring occasionally, or until the chicken and sausage are almost cooked through. Stir in the seasoning mix, tomatoes with their juice and spinach. Cover, reduce the heat to medium-low, and cook for 5 minutes, stirring once, or until the chicken and sausage are cooked through.

PER SERVING: 443 calories, 34g protein, 14g carbohydrates, 28g total fat, 8g saturated fat, 4g fibre, 1,237mg sodium

PEPPERS STUFFED WITH ITALIAN SAUSAGE

PREP TIME: 10 MINUTES | **TOTAL TIME:** 30 MINUTES

Makes 4 servings

While I love stuffed peppers, I don't like the time required to bake them nor the typical use of carbohydrate-rich stuffing contents. So here is a version of stuffed green peppers with some time-saving manoeuvres built in, along with no grains used in the stuffing. This recipe makes enough ultra-saucy mixture to coat shirataki spaghetti or 'riced cauliflower'.

2 tbsp extra-virgin olive oil

450g (1lb) minced Italian sausages

1 small onion, finely chopped

2 garlic cloves, finely chopped

1 tsp Italian Seasoning Mix (page 56)

1 tin (400g/14oz) chopped tomatoes

1 jar (450g/16oz) tomato sauce, divided

4 green peppers, tops and cores removed

1 tbsp water

Preheat the oven to 190°C/375°F/Gas mark 5.

In a large frying pan over a medium heat, heat the oil. Cook the sausage, onion, garlic and seasoning mix for 5 minutes, or until the sausage is browned and the onion is soft. Stir in the tomatoes with their juice and half the sauce, cover, and cook for 5 minutes.

Meanwhile, place the peppers in a microwaveable 23cm (9in) glass pie plate or a 20 x 20cm (8 x 8in) glass baking dish. Add the water, then microwave on high power for 5 minutes, or until the peppers are very soft.

Spoon the sausage mixture into the peppers. Pour the remaining tomato sauce over the peppers. Bake for 10 minutes, or until heated through.

PER SERVING: 318 calories, 22g protein, 21g carbohydrates, 17g total fat, 5g saturated fat, 5g fibre, 1,475mg sodium

PEPPER PIZZAS

PREP TIME: 5 MINUTES | **TOTAL TIME:** 25 MINUTES

Makes 4 servings

This is a variation on the stuffed pepper theme that tastes and smells like pizza! The mixture can be varied in many different ways. For instance, replace the Italian sausage with minced beef or turkey or add Taco Seasoning Mix (page 57).

2 tbsp extra-virgin olive oil

450g (1lb) Italian sausages, loose or finely chopped

375g (13oz) pizza sauce

4 large yellow peppers, halved

4 tbsp water, divided

150g (5oz) grated mozzarella cheese

....

Preheat the oven to 190°C/375°F/Gas mark 5.

In a large frying pan over a medium heat, heat the oil. Cook the sausage, stirring constantly, for 5 minutes, or until browned. Stir in the pizza sauce. Cover and cook for 5 minutes.

Meanwhile, place the peppers in 2 microwaveable 23cm (9in) glass pie plates or 20 x 20cm (8 x 8in) glass baking dishes. Add 1 tablespoon water to each, then microwave separately on high power for 5 minutes, or until the peppers are soft.

Spoon the sausage mixture equally into the peppers. Top with the cheese and bake for 5 minutes, or until the cheese melts.

PER SERVING: 393 calories, 30g protein, 21g carbohydrates, 23g total fat, 8g saturated fat, 5g fibre, 1,290mg sodium

PROVOLONE, PROSCIUTTO AND KALAMATA OLIVE PIZZA

PREP TIME: 10 MINUTES | **TOTAL TIME:** 30 MINUTES

Makes 4 servings

The flavour combinations of this pizza may be better suited to adult palates. A kid-friendly version can be made by replacing prosciutto with sliced salami or sausage and replacing the provolone with additional mozzarella.

PIZZA BASE

285g (10oz) All-Purpose Baking Mix (page 19)

75g (3oz) grated mozzarella cheese

1 egg

2 tbsp extra-virgin olive oil

110g (4oz) water

TOPPING

50g (2oz) provolone, cut into cubes

75g (3oz) grated mozzarella cheese

160g (5oz) pizza sauce (no sugar added)

50g (2oz) prosciutto, cut into 2–3cm (1in) pieces

80g (3oz) pitted Kalamata olives, halved

1 tsp cruched red chillies (optional)

Preheat the oven to 200°C/400°F/Gas mark 6. Line a baking sheet or pizza pan with parchment paper.

To make the crust: In a medium bowl, combine the baking mix and cheese. In a small bowl, mix together the egg, oil and water. Pour into the flour mixture and combine thoroughly.

Lay the dough on the baking sheet or pizza pan and, with moistened hands, press into a 30cm (12in) circle, forming an outer edge. Bake for 10 minutes. Reduce the heat to 180°C/350°F/Gas mark 4.

To make the topping: In a small bowl, combine the provolone and mozzarella. Remove the pizza crust from the oven and top with the sauce, cheese mixture, prosciutto, olives and pepper flakes, if desired. Bake for 10 minutes, or until the cheese melts.

PER SERVING: 703 calories, 31g protein, 24g carbohydrates, 58g total fat, 11g saturated fat, 12g fibre, 1,288mg sodium

MOROCCAN CHICKEN
WITH ROASTED PEPPERS

PREP TIME: 10 MINUTES | **TOTAL TIME:** 30 MINUTES

Makes 4 servings

The exotic combination of seasonings in the Moroccan Seasoning Mix will have your family thinking you slaved over the stove for hours to achieve this unique mixture of flavours, when in reality it took 30 minutes!

1 tbsp Moroccan Seasoning Mix (page 55)

1 tsp sea salt

4 boneless, skinless chicken breast halves

50ml (2fl oz) extra-virgin olive oil, divided

1 onion, quartered and sliced

225g (8oz) chestnut (or baby portobello) mushrooms, quartered

1 jar (200g/7oz) roasted red peppers, drained and cut into 1cm (½in) thick slices

....

In a small bowl, combine the seasoning mix and salt. Rub half the mixture on the chicken breasts.

In a large frying pan over a medium-high heat, heat 2 tablespoons of the oil until hot. Cook the chicken for 5 minutes, turning, or until browned on both sides. Remove to a plate and set aside.

Add the remaining 2 tablespoons oil, the onion, mushrooms and the remaining spice mixture to the pan. Cook for 5 minutes, or until the vegetables are browned.

Add the reserved chicken back to the pan along with the peppers. Reduce the heat to medium-low, cover, and simmer for 10 minutes, or until a thermometer inserted in the thickest portion of the chicken registers 75°C (165°F) and the juices run clear.

PER SERVING: 354 calories, 38g protein, 8g carbohydrates, 19g total fat, 3g saturated fat, 2g fibre, 620mg sodium

SPICY CHICKEN THIGHS

PREP TIME: 5 MINUTES | **TOTAL TIME:** 30 MINUTES

Makes 8 servings

Since chicken wings take longer than 30 minutes to prepare, using boneless thighs allows for all the great flavour in less time. If you prefer a more mellow heat, this recipe also works if you dip the chicken thighs in the sauce mixture before baking. The sauce is also great on chicken wings. Change this recipe by brushing the thighs with Barbecue Sauce (page 35) or Ginger–Miso Sauce (page 37) instead of the butter mixture.

Serve these spicy thighs as they are or with Ranch Dressing (page 45) or a sugar-free blue cheese dressing for dipping.

1.3kg (3lb) boneless, skinless chicken thighs

½ tsp sea salt

½ tsp freshly ground black pepper

50g (2oz) butter, melted

60g (2½oz) hot chilli sauce

Preheat the oven to 220°C/425°F/Gas mark 7.

Place the chicken thighs on a rimmed baking sheet. Sprinkle with the salt and black pepper. Bake for 20 minutes, or until a thermometer inserted in the thickest portion registers 75°C (165°F) and the juices run clear.

Meanwhile, in a large bowl, combine the melted butter and hot chilli sauce. Add the hot chicken and toss to coat.

PER SERVING: 509 calories, 66g protein, 0g carbohydrates, 26g total fat, 11g saturated fat, 0g fibre, 1,072mg sodium

THAI RED CURRY CHICKEN

PREP TIME: 10 MINUTES | **TOTAL TIME:** 30 MINUTES

Makes 4 servings

Thai dishes make use of the wonderful properties of coconut, the unsung hero of the wheat-free world. This Thai Red Curry Chicken can be made as spicy hot as you like by adjusting the quantity of red curry paste you add to the Thai Red Curry Sauce.

For variety, other vegetables can be added or substituted, such as sliced courgettes, sliced carrots or sugar snap peas. Likewise, pork or beef can be substituted for chicken.

2 tbsp coconut oil

675g (1½lb) boneless, skinless chicken breasts, cut into 2–3cm (1in) strips

3 garlic cloves, finely chopped

5 spring onions, chopped

1 red pepper, thinly sliced

110g (4oz) shiitake mushrooms, sliced

1 tin (225g/8oz) sliced bamboo shoots, drained

435g (15oz) Thai Red Curry Sauce (page 36)

15g (½oz) chopped coriander or Thai basil

In a large frying pan over a medium-high heat, heat the oil. Cook the chicken for 5 minutes, or until beginning to brown on all sides, but not completely cooked through. Transfer to a plate and set aside.

Add the garlic, spring onions, pepper, mushrooms and bamboo shoots to the pan. Cook, stirring constantly, for 3 minutes, or until the pepper is lightly browned. Add the reserved chicken, along with accumulated juices and the curry sauce. Stir to partially submerge the chicken in the liquid. Reduce the heat to medium, cover, and cook, stirring occasionally, for 10 minutes, or until the chicken is cooked through. Stir in the coriander or basil.

PER SERVING: 490 calories, 41g protein, 12g carbohydrates, 32g total fat, 25g saturated fat, 4g fibre, 566mg sodium

GINGER–MISO CHICKEN

PREP TIME: 5 MINUTES | **TOTAL TIME:** 20 MINUTES

Makes 4 servings

Preparation time is slashed on this Asian-style chicken rich with the flavours of ginger, miso, wasabi and sesame by using the prepared Ginger–Miso Sauce. Serve alongside steamed spinach or atop shirataki noodles or 'riced' cauliflower.

3 tbsp extra-virgin olive oil
   or coconut oil, divided

675g (1½lb) chicken mini fillets

4 spring onions, sliced

225g (8oz) shiitake mushrooms, sliced

165g (6oz) Ginger–Miso Sauce
   (page 37)

In a large frying pan over a medium-high heat, heat 2 tablespoons of the oil. Cook the chicken for 2 minutes, turning once, or until browned. Work in batches, if necessary. Transfer to a plate and set aside.

Reduce the heat to medium. Add the remaining 1 tablespoon oil to the pan. Cook the spring onions and mushrooms, stirring, for 2 minutes, or until the mushrooms are lightly browned. Place the reserved chicken on top of the vegetables, and pour the ginger sauce over the chicken. Cover and cook for 10 minutes, or until the chicken is no longer pink and the juices run clear.

PER SERVING: 412 calories, 39g protein, 8g carbohydrates, 24g total fat, 3g saturated fat, 3g fibre, 492mg sodium

MAPLE–PECAN CHICKEN

PREP TIME: 10 MINUTES | **TOTAL TIME:** 20 MINUTES

Makes 4 servings

A sweet and crunchy coating makes this quick and easy chicken cutlet recipe a kid-friendly dish.

The ground pecans can be purchased pre-ground or you can simply grind whole nuts in your food processor, food chopper or coffee grinder.

45g (1½oz) ground pecans

¼ tsp sea salt

2 tbsp butter, melted

1 tbsp sugar-free maple-flavoured syrup

450g (1lb) chicken mini fillets

1 tbsp butter

1 tbsp olive oil

....

In a shallow bowl or pie plate, combine the ground pecans and the salt. In a separate shallow bowl or pie plate, combine the 2 tablespoons melted butter and the syrup. Dip each chicken fillet into the butter mixture, evenly coating both sides. Dredge in the pecan mixture, pressing lightly to coat both sides.

In a large frying pan over a medium heat, heat 1 tablespoon butter and the oil until hot. Cook the chicken for 8 minutes, turning once, or until the chicken is no longer pink, and the juices run clear.

PER SERVING: 290 calories, 25g protein, 2g carbohydrates, 20g total fat, 7g saturated fat, 1g fibre, 353mg sodium

160 | MAIN DISHES

BARBECUE BACON-WRAPPED CHICKEN

PREP TIME: 10 MINUTES | **TOTAL TIME:** 25 MINUTES

Makes 4 servings

Quick and easy, this nutritionally complete meal has something to satisfy every family member. The bacon makes the chicken perfectly compatible with breakfast if there are leftovers!

4 boneless, skinless chicken breast halves

12 rashers bacon

110g (4oz) cherry tomatoes, halved

8 spring onions, cut into 5cm (2in) pieces

⅛ tsp sea salt

155g (5½oz) Barbecue Sauce (page 35)

Place the oven rack 15cm (6in) from the heat source and preheat the grill. Line a baking sheet or grill pan with foil.

Wrap 3 rashers of bacon around each chicken breast half and set on the baking sheet or grill pan.

Grill for 6 minutes, or until the bacon begins to crisp and brown. Remove from the oven and turn the chicken over. Scatter the tomatoes and spring onions around the chicken and sprinkle with the salt. Return to the oven and grill for 6 minutes, or until the bacon is cooked through and a thermometer inserted in the thickest portion of the chicken registers 75°C (165°F) and the juices run clear.

Spoon 2 tablespoons of the barbecue sauce over each chicken breast half. Stir the vegetables and grill for 1 minute.

PER SERVING: 545 calories, 45g protein, 11g carbohydrates, 37g total fat, 13g saturated fat, 2g fibre, 875mg sodium

CAJUN CHICKEN CUTLETS

PREP TIME: 5 MINUTES | **TOTAL TIME:** 20 MINUTES

Makes 4 servings

I economize on time with this spicy-hot Cajun chicken dish by using the Cajun Seasoning Mix.

This dish goes exceptionally well over Spinach Gratin.

3 tbsp Mayonnaise (page 40 or shop-bought)

2 tbsp ground almonds/flour

1 tbsp Cajun Seasoning Mix (page 58)

1 tsp Sriracha or hot chilli sauce (optional)

½ tsp sea salt

4 boneless, skinless chicken breast halves

Spinach Gratin (optional, page 128)

....

Preheat the oven to 220°C/425°F/Gas mark 7. Line a baking sheet with parchment paper or foil.

In a small bowl, combine the mayonnaise, ground almonds/flour, seasoning mix, Sriracha or hot-pepper sauce (if desired) and salt.

Place the chicken breasts on the baking sheet and brush the tops evenly with the mayonnaise mixture.

Bake for 15 minutes, or until a thermometer inserted in the thickest portion registers 75°C (165°F) and the juices run clear. If additional browning is desired, grill for 2–3 minutes. If serving with Spinach Gratin, prepare the spinach while the chicken is baking.

PER SERVING: 263 calories, 31g protein, 2g carbohydrates, 14g total fat, 2g saturated fat, 1g fibre, 517mg sodium

CHICKEN PICCATA

PREP TIME: 5 MINUTES | **TOTAL TIME:** 30 MINUTES

Makes 4 servings

The classic *piccata* method of slicing, coating and sautéing meat in a piquant sauce makes a comeback in a wheat-free, healthy version. Olive oil, lemon, capers and butter create that familiar rich Italian flavour that goes so well with steamed green vegetables, mushrooms sautéed in butter or 'riced' cauliflower.

The chicken can be replaced by veal, pork chops, white fish or sliced aubergine.

55g (2oz) ground almonds/flour

¼ tsp sea salt

570g (1¼lb) chicken mini fillets

50ml (2fl oz) extra-virgin olive oil

110ml (4fl oz) chicken stock

1 medium shallot, finely chopped, or
   1 large garlic clove, finely chopped

50ml (2fl oz) lemon juice

2 tbsp capers

3 tbsp unsalted butter, sliced

2 tbsp chopped fresh parsley

In a shallow bowl or pie plate, combine the ground almonds/flour and salt. Dredge the chicken mini fillets in the flour mixture, shaking off any excess.

In a large frying pan over a medium heat, heat the oil until hot. Working in batches if necessary, cook the chicken, for 6 minutes, turning once, or until golden brown and the chicken is no longer pink and the juices run clear. Transfer to a warm platter and cover loosely with foil.

Add the stock and shallot or garlic to the pan, increase the heat to high, and cook, stirring with a wooden spoon or spatula to loosen any browned bits. Boil for 4 minutes, or until the stock has reduced by half. Add the lemon juice and capers and continue simmering for 2 minutes. Remove from the heat and add the butter, stirring until the butter melts and thickens the sauce. Stir in the parsley. Spoon the sauce over the chicken.

PER SERVING: 462 calories, 35g protein, 4g carbohydrates, 34g total fat, 9g saturated fat, 2g fibre, 485mg sodium

CHICKEN PAPRIKA

PREP TIME: 10 MINUTES | **TOTAL TIME:** 30 MINUTES

Makes 4 servings

The flavour of this traditional Hungarian dish is defined by the red pepper and paprika, which highlight the flavour background of chicken, onion and soured cream. Therefore, use the freshest and sweetest red pepper and the best-quality paprika that fits in your budget.

This dish goes well over Courgette Noodles (page 130).

2 tbsp extra-virgin olive oil

1 onion, thinly sliced

1 large red pepper, thinly sliced

675g (1½lb) chicken fillets

2 garlic cloves, finely chopped

2 tbsp smoked paprika

½ tsp sea salt

110ml (4fl oz) chicken stock

225ml (8fl oz) soured cream

In a large frying pan over a medium-high heat, heat the oil until hot. Cook the onion and pepper, stirring frequently, for 5 minutes, or until lightly browned. Add the chicken and cook for 5 minutes, turning, or until browned. Add the garlic, paprika and salt and cook, stirring constantly, for 2 minutes.

Add the stock. Bring to a simmer. Reduce the heat to medium-low, cover and simmer for 5 minutes, or until the chicken is no longer pink and the juices run clear. Stir in the soured cream.

PER SERVING: 396 calories, 39g protein, 10g carbohydrates, 22g total fat, 8g saturated fat, 3g fibre, 481mg sodium

ROASTED RED PEPPER CHICKEN ALFREDO

PREP TIME: 10 MINUTES | **TOTAL TIME:** 25 MINUTES

4 servings

Here is a wheat-free, dairy-free version of chicken in a creamy Alfredo sauce that also folds in the delightful flavour of roasted red pepper.

1 tin (400ml/14fl oz) coconut milk

1 large roasted red pepper (from a jar), roughly chopped

3 packets (225g/8oz each) shirataki fettuccine, rinsed and drained

2 tbsp extra-virgin olive oil

450g (1lb) chicken fillets, cut into 2–3cm (1in) pieces

½ tsp sea salt

3 garlic cloves, finely chopped

50g (2oz) Parmesan cheese, grated

2 tbsp chopped fresh basil

In a blender or food processor, combine the coconut milk and pepper. Blend or process for 1 minute and set aside.

Prepare the fettuccine according to the packet instructions. Drain.

Meanwhile, in a large saucepan over a medium-high heat, heat the oil until hot. Sprinkle the chicken with the salt and cook for 5 minutes, or until the chicken is barely pink. Add the garlic and cook, stirring, for 1 minute. Add the reserved coconut milk mixture.

Heat just until the mixture begins to boil, reduce the heat to medium-low, and simmer for 5 minutes. Stir in the cheese and basil and cook for 2 minutes or until the sauce thickens slightly. Add the fettuccine and toss to coat well.

PER SERVING: 441 calories, 30g protein, 6g carbohydrates, 34g total fat, 22g saturated fat, 2g fibre, 503mg sodium

CAJUN TURKEY BURGERS

PREP TIME: 5 MINUTES | **TOTAL TIME:** 15 MINUTES

Makes 4 burgers

These turkey burgers explode with the spicy flavours of the Cajun Seasoning Mix. If the seasoning is pre-made, these burgers can be on the table in 15 minutes. For a change of pace, substitute any of the other seasoning mixes.

Serve topped with Cheddar cheese, sliced tomato and rocket, either with or without being sandwiched inside Basic Sandwich Muffins (page 27).

450g (1lb) minced turkey

2 tbsp Cajun Seasoning Mix (page 58)

1 tbsp hot chilli sauce (optional)

2 tbsp extra-virgin olive oil or coconut oil

In a large bowl, combine the turkey, seasoning mix and hot chilli sauce (if desired) and mix thoroughly. Form into 4 burgers.

In a large frying pan over a medium heat, heat the oil until hot. Cook the burgers for 8 minutes, turning once, or until a thermometer inserted in the centre registers 75°C (165°F) and the meat is no longer pink.

PER SERVING: 239 calories, 23g protein, 2g carbohydrates, 16g total fat, 3g saturated fat, 1g fibre, 271mg sodium

MISO-GLAZED ORANGE ROUGHY

PREP TIME: 5 MINUTES | **TOTAL TIME:** 20 MINUTES

Makes 4 servings

The tangy Asian flavours of the Ginger–Miso Sauce are put to use to create this fish dish in a snap.

Any white fish can be substituted for the orange roughy, such as cod, haddock, flounder or trout.

675g (1½lb) orange roughy or other white fish fillets

80g (3oz) Ginger–Miso Sauce (page 37)

1 tbsp chopped coriander, for garnish

Preheat the oven to 190°C/375°F/Gas mark 5.

Arrange the fish fillets in a 32 x 23cm (13 x 9in) baking dish. Cover each with the ginger sauce. Bake for 15 minutes, or until the fish flakes easily. Serve sprinkled with the coriander, if desired.

PER SERVING: 136 calories, 20g protein, 1g carbohydrates, 5g total fat, 0.5g saturated fat, 0g fibre, 226mg sodium

CAJUN BAKED FISH WITH PRAWN CREAM SAUCE

PREP TIME: 5 MINUTES | **TOTAL TIME:** 20 MINUTES

Makes 4 servings

The peppery Cajun Seasoning Mix and creamy sauce with prawns liven up the light flavours of any white fish, such as cod, haddock, flounder or orange roughy.

FISH

- 4 cod, haddock or other firm white fish fillets (450g/1lb)
- 2 tbsp butter, melted
- 2 tsp lemon juice
- 1 tsp Cajun Seasoning Mix (page 58)

SAUCE

- 2 tbsp butter, divided
- 110g (4oz) peeled and de-veined medium prawns, chopped
- 2 tbsp snipped chives
- 75g (3oz) cream cheese, cubed
- 225ml (8fl oz) cream
- $\frac{1}{8}$ tsp sea salt

To make the fish: Preheat the oven to 190°C/375°F/Gas mark 5. Grease a 32 × 23cm (13 × 9in) baking dish.

Place the fish fillets in the baking dish. In a small bowl, combine the melted butter, lemon juice and seasoning mix. Brush the butter mixture on the fillets. Bake for 15 minutes, or until the fish flakes easily. While the fish is baking, prepare the prawn cream sauce.

To make the sauce: In a medium frying pan over a medium-high heat, melt 1 tablespoon of the butter. Cook the prawns and chives, stirring frequently, for 2 minutes, or just until the prawns turn pink. Push the prawns towards the outer edges of the pan and reduce the heat to medium-low. Add the remaining 1 tablespoon butter and the cream cheese to the centre of the pan, stirring until softened and melted. Add the cream and salt. Simmer, stirring frequently, for 5 minutes, or until the sauce bubbles gently and thickens. Remove from the heat.

Serve the fillets topped with the prawn cream sauce.

PER SERVING: 407 calories, 27g protein, 4g carbohydrates, 31g total fat, 19g saturated fat, 0g fibre, 483mg sodium

PARMESAN-CRUSTED COD

PREP TIME: 5 MINUTES | **TOTAL TIME:** 20 MINUTES

Makes 4 servings

The combination of grated Parmesan cheese and Italian Seasoning Mix can put any conventional breading to shame!

25g (1oz) Parmesan cheese, grated	675g (1½lb) cod, cut into 4 pieces
½ tsp Italian Seasoning Mix (page 56)	2 tbsp olive oil

Preheat the oven to 190°C/375°F/Gas mark 5.

In a small bowl, combine the cheese and seasoning mix.

Arrange the cod in a 32 x 23cm (13 x 9in) baking dish. Brush with the oil and top with the cheese mixture.

Bake for 15 minutes, or until the fish flakes easily.

PER SERVING: 175 calories, 22g protein, 1g carbohydrates, 9g total fat, 2g saturated fat, 0g fibre, 138mg sodium

FILLET OF FISH AMANDINE

PREP TIME: 10 MINUTES | **TOTAL TIME:** 20 MINUTES

Makes 4 servings

Here's a re-creation of a classic white fish recipe, the sort that just crumbles apart with your fork and bursts open with the heady combined scents and flavours of lemon, butter and fish, with crunch provided by toasted almonds.

Fillet of sole, flounder or other white fish can be substituted for the tilapia.

55g (2oz) ground almonds/flour	3 tbsp extra-virgin olive oil, divided
¼ tsp onion powder	60g (2½oz) slivered almonds
¼ tsp sea salt	1 tbsp butter
⅛ tsp cayenne pepper (optional)	2 tbsp lemon juice
4 tilapia fillets (450g/1lb)	4 lemon wedges

Preheat the oven to 180°C/350°F/Gas mark 4.

In a shallow bowl or pie plate, combine the ground almonds/flour, onion powder, salt and cayenne pepper (if desired). Dredge the fish in the mixture, pressing lightly to evenly coat both sides.

In a large frying pan over a medium-high heat, heat 2 tablespoons of the oil until hot. Cook the fillets (with the thicker parts towards the centre of the pan) for 10 minutes, turning once. Add the remaining 1 tablespoon oil to the pan and cook until the fish flakes easily.

Meanwhile, spread the almonds in a shallow baking dish and bake for 5 minutes, or until golden.

Carefully remove the cooked fillets to a platter. Add the butter to the hot pan and stir in the toasted almonds, tossing to coat with the butter. Add the lemon juice and stir. Spoon the buttered almonds and any remaining pan juices over each fillet. Serve with lemon wedges.

PER SERVING: 354 calories, 26g protein, 6g carbohydrates, 26g total fat, 6g saturated fat, 3g fibre, 215mg sodium

COCONUT-CRUSTED FISH FINGERS

PREP TIME: 10 MINUTES | **TOTAL TIME:** 25 MINUTES

Makes 4 servings

These crunchy coconut-crusted fish fingers are a kid-friendly way to get the family to eat more healthy fish. For a cheesy coating, add a tablespoon of grated Parmesan cheese to the coconut.

Serve with coleslaw or steamed vegetables.

45g (1½oz) unsweetened shredded or desiccated coconut

45g (1½oz) ground golden flaxseeds

½ tsp sea salt

50g (2oz) butter, melted

450g (1lb) cod or haddock fillets, cut into 1 x 8cm (½ x 3in) fingers

Preheat the oven to 200°C/400°F/Gas mark 6. Set a wire rack inside a baking tray and coat with olive oil or coconut oil.

In a shallow bowl or pie plate, combine the coconut, flaxseeds and salt. Place the melted butter in a shallow bowl. Dip the fish fingers in the melted butter, shaking off the excess. Dredge in the coconut mixture, turning to coat. Place on the wire rack. Coat lightly with cooking spray or brush with olive or coconut oil.

Bake for 15 minutes, or until the coating is golden and the fish flakes easily.

PER SERVING: 365 calories, 23g protein, 7g carbohydrates, 27g total fat, 17g saturated fat, 5g fibre, 460mg sodium

SEARED SALMON OVER SESAME SPINACH

PREP TIME: 5 MINUTES | **TOTAL TIME:** 15 MINUTES

Makes 4 servings

Time is saved with this quick but elegant seared salmon recipe by using just one pan. If you're not in a rush, you can steam the spinach separately, drain it, and then add the Ginger–Miso Sauce.

1 tbsp coconut oil

4 salmon steaks (about 225g/8oz each)

350g (6oz each) fresh spinach

165g (6oz) Ginger–Miso Sauce (page 37)

In a large frying pan over a medium-high heat, heat the oil. Cook the salmon steaks for 5 minutes. Turn and top with the spinach. Pour the sesame sauce over the spinach. Cover and cook for 3 minutes, or until the salmon is opaque and the spinach is wilted.

Serve the spinach with the salmon placed on top, drizzled with any pan juices.

PER SERVING: 570calories, 46g protein, 5g carbohydrates, 40g total fat, 10g saturated fat, 2g fibre, 464mg sodium

SALMON CROQUETTES

PREP TIME: 10 MINUTES | **TOTAL TIME:** 20 MINUTES

Makes 4 servings

The lively flavours of the Herbes de Provence bring simple tinned salmon to life in this re-imagined version of fish cakes.

60g (2½oz) Mayonnaise (page 40 or shop-bought)

1 celery stick, finely diced

1 tbsp fresh lemon juice

1 tsp Herbes de Provence (page 59)

¾ tsp mustard powder

2 tins (170g/6oz each) skinless and boneless pink salmon, drained and flaked

1 egg, lightly beaten

65g (2½oz) ground golden flaxseeds

2 tbsp extra-virgin olive oil

8 tsp Garlicky Mayo Spread (page 41)

In a medium bowl, combine the mayonnaise, celery, lemon juice, Herbes de Provence, mustard, salmon, egg and flaxseeds. Mix well. Shape into eight 5cm (2in) patties.

In a large frying pan over a medium heat, heat the oil. Cook the patties for 6 minutes, turning once, or until golden brown. Serve with the mayo spread.

PER SERVING: 404 calories, 20g protein, 5g carbohydrates, 35g total fat, 4g saturated fat, 4g fibre, 437mg sodium

SALMON BURGERS OVER PORTOBELLOS

PREP TIME: 10 MINUTES | **TOTAL TIME:** 20 MINUTES

Makes 4 servings

While these salmon burgers go well on mushrooms, as in the recipe below, they can also be used as part of a sandwich between 2 slices of Basic Focaccia (page 21) with Garlicky Mayo Spread (page 41). For a spicy version, add 1 seeded and finely chopped green chilli to the mixture and use coriander in place of the dill.

4 large portobello mushrooms (10–13cm/4–5in diameter), stems removed

3 tbsp melted coconut oil or extra-virgin olive oil, divided

¾ tsp sea salt, divided

2 spring onions, finely chopped, or ¼ onion, finely chopped

½ roasted red pepper, finely chopped

2 tins (170g/6oz each) skinless and boneless pink salmon, drained and flaked

1 egg, lightly beaten

30g (1¼oz) ground golden flaxseeds

2 tbsp chopped fresh dill

Preheat the oven to 200°C/400°F/Gas mark 6.

Brush the tops of the mushrooms with 1½ tablespoon of the oil and place, stem-side up, on a baking sheet. Drizzle ½ tablespoon of the oil over the gills, and sprinkle with ¼ teaspoon of the salt. Bake for 10 minutes.

Meanwhile, in a medium bowl, combine the spring onions or onion, pepper, salmon, egg, flaxseeds, dill and remaining ½ teaspoon salt. Mix well. Shape into 4 burgers.

In a medium frying pan over a medium heat, heat the remaining 1 tablespoon oil. Cook the burgers for 4 minutes, turning once, or until browned.

Place 1 burger on top of each mushroom. Bake for 5 minutes, or until heated through.

PER SERVING: 258 calories, 20g protein, 7g carbohydrates, 17g total fat, 10g saturated fat, 4g fibre, 570mg sodium

FISH TACOS WITH CHIPOTLE–AVOCADO CREAM

PREP TIME: 10 MINUTES | **TOTAL TIME:** 20 MINUTES

Makes 4 servings

Here's a light 'taco' using lettuce leaves stuffed with a spicy avocado and fish filling. The Tortillas (page 29) or Flaxseed Wraps (page 26) can be used in place of the lettuce.

Chipotle peppers in adobo sauce are smoked ripe jalapeño peppers that are packed in a tomato-based sauce. They have a distinct smoky flavour and can be found online. If you can't find them, you can use chipotle paste. If you prefer a spicier sauce, additional Cajun Seasoning Mix can be added when it is blended; if you prefer a less spicy sauce, reduce the seasoning mix by half.

50g (2oz) butter, melted

2 tinned chipotle peppers in adobo sauce, minced, or chipotle paste, to taste

3 tbsp lime juice, divided

3 tsp freshly grated lime zest, divided

½ tsp sea salt, divided

570g (1¼lb) firm white fish, such as cod, halibut or tilapia, cut into 4 pieces

110ml (4fl oz) soured cream

½ tsp fish seasoning or Cajun Seasoning Mix (page 58)

1 ripe avocado, halved, pitted and peeled

8 medium leaves lettuce (iceberg or romaine)

115g (4oz) finely shredded cabbage

Lime wedges (optional)

In a small bowl, combine the butter, peppers, 1 tablespoon of the lime juice, 2 teaspoons of the lime zest and ¼ teaspoon of the salt until blended. Brush both sides of the fish fillets with the butter mixture. Lightly coat a grill pan or frying pan with cooking spray and heat over a medium-high heat. Cook the fish for 8 minutes, turning once, or until it flakes easily. Transfer to a plate and cover lightly with foil.

Meanwhile, in a blender or small food processor, combine the soured cream, seasoning mix, avocado, the remaining 2 tablespoons lime juice, the remaining 1 teaspoon lime zest and the remaining ¼ teaspoon salt. Blend or process for 30 seconds, or until smooth. Place in a small bowl.

Flake the fish with a fork and place inside the lettuce leaves. Top with the chipotle–avocado cream and shredded cabbage. Serve with lime wedges, if desired.

PER SERVING: 384 calories, 28g protein, 10g carbohydrates, 27g total fat, 13g saturated fat, 4g fibre, 428mg sodium

CARIBBEAN PRAWNS AND RICE

PREP TIME: 10 MINUTES | **TOTAL TIME:** 25 MINUTES

Makes 4 servings

I use the Cajun Seasoning Mix in this quick and easy dish, but bring in the exotic Caribbean combination of ginger, coriander and lime.

½ large head cauliflower, broken into florets

2 tbsp extra-virgin olive oil

4 spring onions, sliced

1 red pepper, thinly sliced

1 tin (400g/14oz) chopped tomatoes

1 tsp Cajun Seasoning Mix (page 58)

2 tbsp grated fresh ginger or 2 tsp ground ginger

450g (1lb) peeled and de-veined medium prawns, tails removed

Juice of 1 small lime

2 tbsp coarsely chopped coriander

Using a food processor with a shredding disk attachment or the largest holes of a box grater, grate the cauliflower. Place the grated cauliflower in a microwaveable bowl. Cover and microwave on high power for 4 minutes, stirring once, or until the desired doneness. Set aside.

In a large frying pan over a medium-high heat, heat the oil. Cook the spring onions and pepper, stirring frequently, for 5 minutes, or until lightly browned. Stir in the tomatoes, seasoning mix and ginger. Cook for 1 minute, or until simmering. Add the prawns, cover, and cook for 3 minutes, or until the prawns are opaque.

Stir in the reserved 'riced' cauliflower, lime juice and coriander. Cook for 2 minutes or until heated through.

PER SERVING: 206 calories, 18g protein, 14g carbohydrates, 9g total fat, 1g saturated fat, 3g fibre, 917mg sodium

PRAWN-STUFFED TOMATOES

PREP TIME: 15 MINUTES | **TOTAL TIME:** 15 MINUTES

Makes 4 servings

Lime and avocado mingle with the flavours of tomato to make an interesting way to enjoy prawns. For the fullest flavour, choose vine-ripened tomatoes, if available.

450g (1lb) frozen cooked medium prawns, thawed

6 large tomatoes, halved lengthwise

60g (2½oz) Mayonnaise (page 40 or shop-bought)

1 celery stick, finely chopped

2 spring onions, thinly sliced

1 tbsp lime juice

¼ tsp sea salt

1 large ripe avocado, halved, pitted, peeled and chopped

Rinse the prawns, pat completely dry with kitchen paper and chop coarsely. Using a spoon, scoop out the flesh of each tomato half and discard.

In a medium bowl, whisk together the mayonnaise, celery, spring onions, lime juice and salt. Add the prawns and toss to coat. Gently fold in the avocado. Divide the mixture among the tomatoes.

PER SERVING: 258 calories, 17g protein, 9g carbohydrates, 18g total fat, 2g saturated fat, 4g fibre, 846mg sodium

CREAMY PRAWNS MARINARA

PREP TIME: 5 MINUTES | **TOTAL TIME:** 25 MINUTES

Makes 4 servings

Humans were meant to eat shellfish!

Here's a way to enjoy prawns that just about anybody can appreciate, kids on up. The prawns go wonderfully with Courgette Noodles, but shirataki noodles or 'riced' cauliflower are other options. A dairy-free version can be made by replacing the double cream with tinned coconut milk. For some added kick, sprinkle the finished dish with ½ teaspoon crushed red chillies.

1 tbsp extra-virgin olive oil

1 shallot, finely chopped

3 garlic cloves, finely chopped

2 tins (400g/14oz each) chopped tomatoes

2 tbsp tomato purée

1 tsp Italian Seasoning Mix (page 56)

1lb (450g) peeled and de-veined large prawns, tails removed

110ml (4fl oz) double cream or tinned coconut milk

Courgette Noodles (page 130), optiona

In a large frying pan, heat the oil over a medium heat. Cook the shallot and garlic for 2 minutes, stirring occasionally. Stir in the tomatoes, tomato purée and seasoning mix and bring to a simmer. Reduce the heat to low and simmer for 10 minutes, stirring occasionally.

Add the prawns, cover and simmer for 3 minutes, or until opaque. Stir in the cream or coconut milk and cook for 2 minutes or until heated through. Serve over courgette noodles, if desired.

PER SERVING: 293 calories, 20g protein, 19g carbohydrates, 16g total fat, 8g saturated fat, 4g fibre, 981mg sodium

CHORIZO-PRAWN TORTILLAS

PREP TIME: 10 MINUTES | **TOTAL TIME:** 20 MINUTES

Makes 4 servings

The seemingly disparate spiciness of chorizo; the ocean flavours of prawns; and the cool, fresh scent of coriander come together deliciously in these easy tortillas.

This recipe's already quick, but you can save even more time by chopping the garlic and onion in the food processor. If you want to skip the tortillas altogether, add 'riced' cauliflower when you add the prawns to make an easy version of paella.

2 tbsp extra-virgin olive oil

1 onion, finely chopped

2 garlic cloves, finely chopped

170–225g (6–8oz) chorizo sausage, thinly sliced

450g (1lb) peeled and de-veined small to medium prawns, tails removed

2 tbsp Taco Seasoning Mix (page 57)

2 tbsp chopped coriander

4 Tortillas (page 29)

In a large frying pan over a medium heat, heat the oil. Cook the onion and garlic for 3 minutes, stirring constantly, or until softened.

Add the chorizo and cook for 5 minutes, stirring occasionally, or until cooked through. Add the prawns and seasoning mix. Cook for 2 minutes, stirring frequently, or until opaque. Stir in the coriander. Spoon over the tortillas.

PER SERVING: 405 calories, 29g protein, 18g carbohydrates, 26g total fat, 4g saturated fat, 8g fibre, 998mg sodium

INDIAN CURRY PRAWNS

PREP TIME: 5 MINUTES | **TOTAL TIME:** 15 MINUTES

Makes 4 servings

The fragrant and exotic scents of the curry in a thick coconut milk base create a wonderful way to enjoy seafood. To save even more time (and transform this into a Thai curry dish), skip the ginger, garlic and curry powder and use 1 cup Thai Red Curry Sauce (page 36) in place of the coconut milk. Either way, try serving over 'riced' cauliflower.

3 tbsp coconut oil or ghee

1 onion, thinly sliced

1 tsp finely chopped fresh ginger

1 tsp finely chopped garlic

4 tsp curry powder

½ tsp sea salt

225ml (8fl oz) tinned coconut milk

675g (1½lb) peeled and de-veined medium prawns, tails removed

2 tbsp chopped coriander

In a large frying pan over a medium heat, heat the oil or ghee. Cook the onion for 5 minutes, or until lightly browned. Stir in the ginger, garlic, curry powder and salt and cook for 1 minute. Add the coconut milk and bring to a simmer. Add the prawns and cook for 2 minutes, or until opaque. Remove from the heat and stir in the coriander.

PER SERVING: 301 calories, 17g protein, 7g carbohydrates, 24g total fat, 20g saturated fat, 2g fibre, 849mg sodium

PRAWN SCAMPI

PREP TIME: 10 MINUTES | **TOTAL TIME:** 20 MINUTES

Makes 4 servings

Classic prawn scampi returns, free of the tyranny of the wheat noodle! While the prawn scampi alone can be served alongside some steamed asparagus or fresh mushrooms sautéed in butter, serve it with shirataki noodles to mimic the classic Italian dish.

3 tbsp extra-virgin olive oil, divided

75g (3oz) fresh mushrooms, sliced

3 tbsp butter, divided

675g (1½lb) peeled and de-veined large prawns, tails removed

5 garlic cloves, finely chopped

1 tsp Italian Seasoning Mix (page 56)

3 tbsp lemon juice

2 tbsp dry white wine or chicken stock

2 tbsp finely chopped fresh parsley

Cooked shirataki noodles (optional)

In a large frying pan over a medium-high heat, heat 1 tablespoons of the oil until hot. Cook the mushrooms for 5 minutes, stirring occasionally, or until lightly browned and their moisture is released. Transfer to a bowl and set aside.

Add the remaining 2 tablespoons oil and 1 tablespoon of the butter to the same pan and heat over a medium-high heat to melt the butter. Cook the prawns for 2 minutes, stirring frequently, or just until opaque (do not overcook). Transfer to the bowl with the mushrooms.

Reduce the heat to medium. Melt 1 tablespoon of the butter in the frying pan. Add the garlic and cook for 1 minute, stirring constantly. Add the remaining 1 tablespoon butter to the pan along with the seasoning mix. Whisk in the lemon juice and wine or stock and cook for 1 minute, whisking constantly. Return the reserved prawns and mushrooms, along with accumulated juices, to the pan. Cook for 1 minute or until heated through. Stir in the parsley. Serve over shirataki noodles, if desired.

PER SERVING: 318 calories, 24g protein, 5g carbohydrates, 21g total fat, 7g saturated fat, 0.5g fibre, 1,043mg sodium

EASY BAKED SCALLOPS

PREP TIME: 10 MINUTES | **TOTAL TIME:** 25 MINUTES

Makes 4 servings

Here's a good, old-fashioned recipe for baked scallops dripping with butter, but with no sign of wheat! We replace breadcrumbs with a mixture of ground almonds/flour and Parmesan cheese that re-creates that buttery, crumbly topping that many wheat-free people miss.

25g (1oz) ground almonds/flour

25g (1oz) Parmesan cheese, finely grated

1 tsp fish seasoning or Moroccan Seasoning Mix (page 48), divided

450g (1lb) medium sea scallops, rinsed and patted dry

2 tbsp lemon juice

2 tbsp butter, melted

....

Preheat the oven to 190°C/375°F/Gas mark 5. Grease a 28 x 18cm (11 x 7in) baking dish.

In a shallow bowl or dish, combine the ground almonds/flour, cheese and ½ teaspoon of the seasoning mix. Dredge the scallops in the cheese mixture, pressing to coat evenly. Place on the baking dish.

In a small bowl, combine the lemon juice, butter and the remaining ½ teaspoon seasoning mix. Carefully drizzle over the scallops to keep the topping intact.

Bake for 12 minutes, or until just barely opaque. Turn the oven to grill and cook for 2 minutes, or until lightly browned on top.

PER SERVING: 197 calories, 17g protein, 7g carbohydrates, 12g total fat, 5g saturated fat, 1g fibre, 677mg sodium

CURRIED VEGETABLES

PREP TIME: 10 MINUTES | **TOTAL TIME:** 30 MINUTES

Makes 4 servings

These flavourful Indian curried vegetables can stand alone as a main meal or serve as a substantial side dish. The vegetables are easily varied; try using sliced carrots, baby onions, spring onions or broccoli.

2 tbsp coconut oil

1 onion, chopped

2 garlic cloves, finely chopped

500g (1lb 2oz) small frozen cauliflower florets, thawed, or fresh

300g (11oz) frozen spinach, thawed, or 180g (6½oz) fresh spinach

1 large tomato, chopped

435g (15oz) Thai Red Curry Sauce (page 36)

¼ tsp sea salt

15g (½oz) coarsely chopped coriander

In a large frying pan over a medium-high heat, heat the oil. Cook the onion and garlic for 3 minutes. Stir in the cauliflower, cover, and cook for 7 minutes, stirring occasionally. Add the spinach, tomato, curry sauce and salt. Cover and simmer for 10 minutes, or until the cauliflower is soft. Stir in the coriander.

PER SERVING: 311 calories, 5g protein, 15g carbohydrates, 28g total fat, 24g saturated fat, 5g fibre, 493mg sodium

SPANAKOPITA BURGERS

PREP TIME: 15 MINUTES | **TOTAL TIME:** 30 MINUTES

4 servings

This is a variation on spanakopita, or Greek spinach pie, that includes all of the wonderful flavourful ingredients – spinach, feta cheese, onion and egg – but without the unhealthy effects of the pastry. Here it is re-created as a burger that can be eaten as is or sandwiched between two slices of Sandwich Bread (page 20) or Basic Focaccia (page 21).

3 tbsp extra-virgin olive oil, divided

1 small onion, finely chopped

570g (1lb 4oz) frozen chopped spinach, thawed and squeezed dry

1 tsp dried oregano

½ tsp garlic salt

½ tsp freshly ground black pepper

2 tsp fresh lemon juice

150g (5oz) feta cheese, crumbled

1 egg, lightly beaten

65g (2½oz) ground golden flaxseeds

In a large frying pan over a medium-high heat, heat 1 tablespoon of the oil. Cook the onion for 3 minutes, stirring frequently, or until lightly browned. Add the spinach and cook for 1 minute, stirring, or until heated through. Transfer to a medium bowl and allow to cool slightly. Add the oregano, garlic salt, pepper, lemon juice, cheese, egg and flaxseeds. Mix to combine. Shape into 4 burgers.

In the pan over a medium heat, heat the remaining 2 tablespoons oil. Cook the burgers for 7 minutes, turning once, or until light brown.

PER SERVING: 322 calories, 12g protein, 13g carbohydrates, 24g total fat, 7g saturated fat, 6g fibre, 670mg sodium

KALE, ONION AND GOAT'S CHEESE PIZZA

PREP TIME: 10 MINUTES | **TOTAL TIME:** 30 MINUTES

Makes 4 servings

The unique mix of flavours in this pizza, best suited to adult palates, elevates a casual dish to the level of something special!

PIZZA DOUGH

285g (10oz) All-Purpose Baking Mix (page 19)

75g (3oz) grated mozzarella cheese

¼ tsp sea salt

1 egg

2 tbsp extra-virgin olive oil

110ml (4fl oz) water

TOPPING

2 tbsp extra-virgin olive oil

280g (10oz) fresh or frozen kale, thawed, torn into small pieces

1 onion, cut into wedges

¼ tsp sea salt

160g (5½oz) pizza sauce (no sugar added)

50g (2oz) goat's cheese, crumbled

Preheat the oven to 200°C/400°F/Gas mark 6. Line a baking sheet or pizza pan with parchment paper.

To make the dough: In a medium bowl, combine the baking mix, cheese and salt. In a small bowl, mix together the egg, oil and water. Pour into the flour mixture and combine thoroughly.

Place the dough on the baking sheet or pizza pan and, with moistened hands, press into a 30cm (12in) circle, forming an outer edge. Bake for 10 minutes. Remove from the oven and set aside. Reduce the heat to 180°C/350°F/Gas mark 4.

To make the topping: Meanwhile, in a large frying pan over a medium heat, heat the oil. Add the kale, onion and salt and cook for 5 minutes, stirring frequently, or until the kale wilts and the onion is soft.

Top the pizza dough with the sauce, kale mixture and goat's cheese. Return to the oven for 10 minutes, or until the cheese melts.

PER SERVING: 698 calories, 27g protein, 30g carbohydrates, 57g total fat, 9g saturated fat, 14g fibre, 1,015mg sodium

PALAK PANEER

PREP TIME: 10 MINUTES | **TOTAL TIME:** 30 MINUTES

Makes 4 servings

This Indian/Pakistani dish serves up a walloping quantity of healthy spinach in an exotic curry sauce.

350g (12oz) baby spinach

2 tbsp ghee or coconut oil

350g (12oz) paneer cheese, cut into 2–3cm (1in) cubes

1 onion, finely chopped

2 garlic cloves, finely chopped

2 tbsp Moroccan Seasoning Mix (page 48)

½ tsp sea salt

1 tin (400g/14oz) chopped tomatoes or 1 tomato, chopped

110ml (4fl oz) tinned coconut milk or cream

....

Place the spinach in a colander set in the sink. Carefully pour 1 litre (1 quart) boiling water over it to wilt the spinach. Set aside to drain.

In a large frying pan over a medium heat, heat the ghee or oil. Cook the cheese for 8 minutes, turning, or until browned. Remove from the pan and set aside on a plate.

In the same pan, cook the onion and garlic for 3 minutes, or until lightly browned. Add the seasoning mix and salt and stir for 1 minute. Add the reserved spinach, the tomatoes and coconut milk or cream. Bring to a simmer. Reduce the heat to medium-low, cover, and simmer for 5 minutes.

Carefully pour the contents of the pan into a food processor and process for 1 minute, or until the spinach and tomatoes are broken down and the mixture is creamy. Return to the pan, add the reserved cheese and heat through.

PER SERVING: 475 calories, 23g protein, 20g carbohydrates, 35g total fat, 24g saturated fat, 6g fibre, 567mg sodium

CHILLIES RELLENOS MINI CASSEROLES

PREP TIME: 5 MINUTES | **TOTAL TIME:** 30 MINUTES

Makes 4 servings

If you're in the mood for something Mexican besides a burrito, here's a nice little option that is deceptively filling and delicious.

4 eggs

175ml (6fl oz) double cream

1 tin or jar (200g/7oz) diced green chillies, drained

185g (6½oz) Cheddar cheese, grated, divided

4 tbsp tomato salsa (optional)

Preheat the oven to 200°C/400°F/Gas mark 6. Grease 4 (225–250g/8–9oz) ramekins and place on a baking sheet.

In a medium bowl, whisk together the eggs and cream. Add the chillies and two-thirds of the cheese and whisk to combine. Divide evenly among the ramekins. Top with the remaining cheese. Bake for 25 minutes, or until a knife inserted in the centre comes out clean. Top each with 1 tablespoon salsa, if desired.

PER SERVING: 406 calories, 17g protein, 5g carbohydrates, 35g total fat, 20g saturated fat, 1g fibre, 468mg sodium

KID-FRIENDLY

FETTUCCINE WITH BASIL-WALNUT PESTO

PREP TIME: 5 MINUTES | **TOTAL TIME:** 15 MINUTES

Makes 2 servings

Bring the magical combination of basil and extra-virgin olive oil together in this simple pasta dish.

Save time by using prepared basil pesto from the recipe on page 31 or shop-bought.

50g (2oz) fresh basil

25g (1oz) walnuts

3 garlic cloves, chopped

75ml (3fl oz) extra-virgin olive oil

25g (1oz) Pecorino cheese, grated

¼ tsp sea salt

2 tsp fresh lemon juice

2 packets (225g/8oz each) shirataki fettuccine noodles, rinsed and drained

In a food chopper or food processor, combine the basil, walnuts and garlic. Chop or process into a paste. Add the oil, cheese, salt and lemon juice and chop or process until the mixture is blended and the pesto is bright green. Set aside.

Prepare the noodles according to the packet instructions. Transfer to a serving bowl.

Top the noodles with the reserved basil mixture and toss to coat well.

PER SERVING: 498 calories, 9g protein, 14g carbohydrates, 48g total fat, 7g saturated fat, 8g fibre, 403mg sodium

SPAGHETTI WITH OLIVES, CAPERS AND GARLIC

PREP TIME: 10 MINUTES | **TOTAL TIME:** 20 MINUTES

Makes 2 servings

This simple 'pasta' dish can serve as a filling main course or a substantial side dish. Don't let the apparent small servings fool you: remember that, minus the appetite-stimulating effects of the gliadin protein of wheat, appetites are satisfied with much less. And this pasta, unlike those made with conventional ingredients or the awful gluten-free flours, does not result in sky-high blood sugars or other distortions of metabolism.

50ml (2fl oz) extra-virgin olive oil

3 garlic cloves, finely chopped

3 spring onions, sliced

¼ tsp sea salt

2 tsp capers

45g (1½oz) pitted Kalamata olives, sliced

2 packets (225g/8oz each) shirataki fettuccine noodles, rinsed and drained

25g (1oz) Parmesan cheese, grated

In a medium frying pan over a medium heat, heat the oil. Cook the garlic, spring onions and salt for 3 minutes, or until the spring onions begin to soften. Stir in the capers and olives. Set aside.

Prepare the noodles according to the packet instructions. Transfer to a serving bowl. Top with the reserved olive mixture and toss to coat. Sprinkle with the cheese.

PER SERVING: 425 calories, 5g protein, 9g carbohydrates, 41g total fat, 7g saturated fat, 1g fibre, 1,142mg sodium

JAPANESE AUBERGINE STIR-FRY

PREP TIME: 15 MINUTES | **TOTAL TIME:** 30 MINUTES

Makes 4 servings

I've served this Japanese aubergine as both a main dish and a substantial side dish alongside beef that had been marinated and sautéed in a (gluten-free) teriyaki sauce. Optionally, 450g (1lb) of finely sliced beef or pork or prawns can be combined with the aubergine itself. (Meat or prawns should be cooked separately, then combined.) If noodles are desired, shirataki would be perfect. Long, thin Asian aubergines can be found in most Asian stores and in some supermarkets.

3 tbsp sesame oil, divided

675g (1½lb) Asian aubergines, quartered lengthwise and sliced 1cm (½in) thick

6 spring onions, sliced

4 garlic cloves, finely chopped

3 tbsp gluten-free soy sauce

2 tbsp grated fresh ginger

50ml (2fl oz) water

25g (1oz) coriander, coarsely chopped

2 tsp sesame seeds

In a large frying pan over a medium heat, heat 2 tablespoons of the oil. Add the aubergine, cover and cook for 10 minutes, stirring occasionally, or until softened.

Add the remaining 1 tablespoon oil. Stir in the spring onions, garlic, soy sauce, ginger and water. Cover and simmer for 5 minutes, stirring occasionally, or until the aubergine is completely soft. Just before serving, stir in the coriander and sprinkle with the sesame seeds.

PER SERVING: 160 calories, 4g protein, 14g carbohydrates, 11g total fat, 1.5g saturated fat, 5g fibre, 669mg sodium

BROCCOLI-CHEESE CASSEROLE

PREP TIME: 10 MINUTES | **TOTAL TIME:** 30 MINUTES

Makes 4 servings

This simple casserole can serve as either a main dish or a substantial side dish alongside pork chops, baked chicken or any form of beef. Other vegetables, such as fresh asparagus or green beans, can be added or can replace the broccoli.

350g (12oz) broccoli florets

110ml (4fl oz) water

2 eggs

125g (4½oz) mature Cheddar cheese, grated, divided

110ml (4fl oz) double cream

35g (1¼oz) ground almonds/flour

½ tsp mustard powder

¼ tsp onion powder

¼ tsp sea salt

Dash of cayenne pepper (optional)

Preheat the oven to 200°C/400°F/Gas mark 6. Grease a 20 x 20cm (8 x 8in) baking dish.

In a microwaveable bowl, place the broccoli florets and water, cover, and microwave on high power for 3 minutes, or until the broccoli is bright green and softened. Drain and place in the baking dish.

In a medium bowl, combine the eggs, half the cheese, the cream, ground almonds/flour, mustard, onion powder, salt and cayenne pepper (if desired). Pour over the broccoli. Top with the remaining cheese.

Bake for 20 minutes, or until a knife inserted in the centre comes out clean.

PER SERVING: 332 calories, 15g protein, 8g carbohydrates, 28g total fat, 14g saturated fat, 4g fibre, 249mg sodium

DESSERTS AND SNACKS

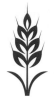

COCONUT–CHOCOLATE TART

PREP TIME: 5 MINUTES | **TOTAL TIME:** 20 MINUTES + CHILLING TIME

Makes 8 servings

Shredded coconut makes a sturdy and delicious pastry case. Here I fill a coconut case with a rich chocolate cream to make a delightful tart appropriate for celebrations or an extra-special dessert.

115g (4oz) shredded or desiccated unsweetened coconut

3 tbsp All-Purpose Baking Mix (page 19)

Sweetener equivalent to 115g (4oz) sugar

3 tbsp coconut oil or butter, melted

400ml (14fl oz) tinned coconut milk

225g (8oz) plain (85% cocoa) chocolate, chopped

½ tsp vanilla extract

¼ tsp almond extract

Preheat the oven to 180°C/350°F/Gas mark 4. Grease a 23cm (9in) pie plate.

In a medium bowl, combine the coconut, baking mix, sweetener equivalent to 3 tablespoons of sugar and the oil or butter and mix thoroughly. Press into the pie plate and bake for 10 minutes, or until the edges are lightly browned. Remove and cool.

Meanwhile, in a medium saucepan over a medium-high heat, heat the coconut milk just until bubbles begin to form. Remove from the heat, add the chocolate, and stir until melted. Stir in the vanilla, almond extract and the remaining sweetener until blended. Pour into the coconut case. Refrigerate until set, at least 1 hour.

PER SERVING: 453 calories, 7g protein, 14g carbohydrates, 46g total fat, 36g saturated fat, 8g fibre, 28mg sodium

BERRY-COCONUT MINI CHEESECAKES

PREP TIME: 10 MINUTES | **TOTAL TIME:** 30 MINUTES + COOLING TIME

Makes 12 cakes

All doubts over how delicious a wheat-free lifestyle can be will crumble with these delicious mini cheesecakes!

I top these with fresh berries, but you can substitute with a drizzle of dark chocolate, a sprinkle of cocoa powder or some more coconut.

145g (5oz) All-Purpose Baking Mix (page 19)

Sweetener equivalent to 115g (4oz) sugar

3 tbsp coconut oil or butter, melted

350g (12oz) cream cheese, at room temperature

125g (4½oz) soured cream or plain Greek yoghurt

2 eggs

15g (½oz) shredded or desiccated unsweetened coconut

330g (11½oz) fresh mixed berries

Preheat the oven to 180°C/350°F/Gas mark 4. Place paper cases in a 12-cup muffin tin.

In a large bowl, combine the baking mix, sweetener equivalent to 1 tablespooon sugar and the coconut oil or butter. Mix thoroughly. Divide among the muffin cups. Press flat in the bottom of each cup with a spoon or your fingers. Set aside.

In a large bowl, with an electric mixer, blend the cream cheese and the remaining sweetener until smooth. Stir in the soured cream or yoghurt. Add the eggs, one at a time, mixing until thoroughly incorporated. Stir in the coconut and mix thoroughly. Divide the batter among the muffin cups. Bake for 20 minutes, or until a knife inserted in the centre comes out clean. (The cheesecakes will puff up during baking and then fall as they cool.)

Allow to cool in the muffin tin for 5 minutes. Remove to a rack to cool completely. Serve each topped with 2 tablespoons of berries.

PER CHEESECAKE: 265 calories, 6g protein, 16g carbohydrates, 22g total fat, 11g saturated fat, 3g fibre, 166mg sodium

CINNAMON DOUGHNUTS

PREP TIME: 10 MINUTES | **TOTAL TIME:** 20 MINUTES + COOLING TIME

Makes 12 doughnuts

An unusual technique is used to create these mini-doughnuts. The result: delicious, bite-sized, *healthy* snacks! Because these doughnuts, unlike conventional wheat flour/sugary/fried doughnuts, are without adverse health implications, you can have them for breakfast, snacks or dessert without worry.

Optionally, you can drizzle the Chocolate Glaze (page 214) or Vanilla Glaze (page 215) over the top.

30g (1¼oz) ground golden flaxseeds

225ml (8fl oz) cold water

85g (3oz) coconut flour

45g (1½oz) shredded or desiccated unsweetened coconut

Sweetener equivalent to 115g (4oz) sugar

1½ tsp ground cinnamon

½ tsp bicarbonate of soda

110ml (4fl oz) coconut oil, melted

1 egg

Preheat the oven to 190°C/375°F/Gas mark 5. Grease a doughnut pan.

In a small mug or bowl, stir together the flaxseeds and water, then place it in the freezer for 5 minutes.

In a large bowl, combine the coconut flour, coconut, sweetener, cinnamon and bicarbonate of soda, and mix. Stir in the coconut oil until well mixed.

Remove the flaxseeds from the freezer and whisk in the egg. Pour the flaxseed mixture into the coconut mixture and mix. Spoon the mixture into the doughnut pan, pressing into the dips, if necessary.

Bake for 10 minutes, or until the doughnuts are slightly firm to the touch and the edges are golden. Allow to cool in the pan for 5 minutes before inverting onto a wire rack to cool completely.

PER DOUGHNUT: 189 calories, 2g protein, 15g carbohydrates, 15g total fat, 12g saturated fat, 5g fibre, 61mg sodium

MINI CHOCOLATE ÉCLAIRS

PREP TIME: 10 MINUTES | **TOTAL TIME:** 30 MINUTES + COOLING TIME

Makes 8 éclairs

Yes: chocolate éclairs! But these are actually healthy. For a more luxurious topping, try the Chocolate Glaze on page 214.

110ml (4fl oz) tinned coconut milk, well stirred

60g (2½oz) butter

30g (1¼oz) coconut flour

2 tsp ground psyllium seeds

⅛ tsp sea salt

2 eggs, at room temperature

225g (8oz) double cream

Sweetener equivalent to 2 tbsp sugar

½ tsp vanilla extract

1 bar (100g/3½oz) dark chocolate (70–85% cocoa), chopped and melted

Preheat the oven to 190°C/375°F/Gas mark 5. Line a baking sheet with parchment paper.

In a medium saucepan over a medium heat, bring the coconut milk and butter to the boil. Remove from the heat and add the flour, psyllium seeds and salt all at once. Stir until incorporated. Return the saucepan to the heat and stir until the mixture pulls together into a loose ball. Remove from the heat and continue stirring for 1 minute, to cool the mixture slightly. Add the eggs, one at a time, stirring to thoroughly incorporate. Stir until the mixture is mostly smooth and takes on a slight sheen.

Spoon or pipe the mixture into eight 5 to 8cm (2 to 3in) lines on the baking sheet. Bake for 20 minutes, or until golden and slightly firm. Remove to a wire rack to cool completely.

Meanwhile, in a large bowl, with an electric mixer on a high speed, beat the cream until stiff peaks form. With the mixer on a low speed, blend in the sweetener and vanilla. Set aside.

Slice each éclair puff in half, and remove the centre dough. Dollop the whipped cream mixture onto the bottom halves. Replace the tops. Drizzle the chocolate over the tops.

PER ÉCLAIR: 280 calories, 4g protein, 10g carbohydrates, 26g total fat, 17g saturated fat, 4g fibre, 116mg sodium

DOUBLE CHOCOLATE MINI CAKES

PREP TIME: 5 MINUTES | **TOTAL TIME:** 30 MINUTES

Makes 4 cakes

Kids love having their own little cakes. These 8cm (3in) mini cakes are just the right size for a filling and healthy celebration.

If a fine cake texture is desired, substitute the baking mix with almond flour from blanched almonds. Optionally, Chocolate Glaze (page 214) or Chocolate Icing (page 217) can be added for *triple* chocolate mini cakes.

145g (5oz) All-Purpose Baking Mix
    (page 19)

2 tbsp unsweetened
    cocoa powder

Sweetener equivalent to
    170g (6oz) sugar

50g (2oz) dark chocolate chips

1 tsp distilled white vinegar

6 tbsp coconut milk (tinned or carton)
    or milk

½ tbsp black treacle

1 egg, beaten

Preheat the oven to 190°C/375°F/Gas mark 5. Grease four 110g (4oz) ramekins.

In a large bowl, combine the baking mix, cocoa, sweetener and chocolate chips. Mix well.

Stir in the vinegar and coconut milk or milk. Allow to stand for 1 minute. Stir in the black treacle and egg, mixing thoroughly. The batter should be the consistency of conventional cake batter, but if it's too thick, add more coconut milk or milk, 1 tablespoon at a time, until the desired thickness is achieved.

Divide the batter among the ramekins. Arrange on a baking sheet and bake for 25 minutes, or until a wooden cocktail stick inserted in the centre of a cake comes out clean.

PER CAKE: 371 calories, 12g protein, 21g carbohydrates, 30g total fat, 10g saturated fat, 9g fibre, 195mg sodium

198 | DESSERTS AND SNACKS

KEY LIME CUPCAKES

PREP TIME: 5 MINUTES | **TOTAL TIME:** 25 MINUTES + COOLING TIME

Makes 12 cupcakes

If your kids love the sharp, tart flavour of limes like mine do, then these Key Lime Cupcakes are sure to satisfy! Modify the tartness simply by increasing or decreasing the amount of lime juice. For an extra-light cake texture, substitute the baking mix with almond flour from blanched almonds.

CUPCAKES

460g (1lb) All-Purpose Baking Mix (page 19)

Sweetener equivalent to 230g (8oz) sugar

½ tsp sea salt

225ml (8fl oz) lime juice

3 eggs

ICING

230g (8oz) cream cheese, at room temperature

Sweetener equivalent to 115g (4oz) sugar

2 tsp lime juice

Preheat the oven to 180°C/350°F/Gas mark 4. Place paper cases in a 12-cup muffin tin.

To make the cupcakes: In a large bowl, combine the baking mix, sweetener and salt. Mix well. Stir in the lime juice and allow to stand for 1 minute. Whisk the eggs and stir into the mixture.

Divide the batter among the muffin cups. Bake for 20 minutes, or until a wooden cocktail stick inserted in the centre of a cupcake comes out clean.

To make the icing: In a small bowl, combine the cream cheese, sweetener and lime juice. Mix well. Spread over the tops of the cooled cupcakes.

PER CUPCAKE: 299 calories, 11g protein, 13g carbohydrates, 25g total fat, 5g saturated fat, 6g fibre, 350mg sodium

PISTACHIO-GREEN TEA CUPCAKES

PREP TIME: 10 MINUTES | **TOTAL TIME:** 30 MINUTES + COOLING TIME

Makes 12 cupcakes

If you love green tea and the health benefits it provides, the ground powder from green tea leaves is a little-known way to obtain them. The green tea powder can be purchased already ground, usually from the matcha variety, or it can be ground from dried green tea leaves.

CUPCAKES

460g (1lb) All-Purpose Baking Mix (page 19)

Sweetener equivalent to 230g (8oz) sugar

110g (4oz) raw pistachios, finely chopped

½ tsp sea salt

2 tsp lemon juice or white vinegar

225ml (8fl oz) buttermilk

50ml (2fl oz) coconut oil, melted

3 eggs

ICING

230g (8oz) cream cheese, at room temperature

Sweetener equivalent to 115g (4oz) sugar

2 tsp green tea powder

½ tsp ground cardamom

Preheat the oven to 180°C/350°F/Gas mark 4. Place paper cases in a 12-cup muffin tin.

To make the cupcakes: In a large bowl, combine the baking mix, sweetener, pistachios and salt. Stir in the lemon juice or vinegar and allow to stand for 1 minute. In a separate bowl, combine the buttermilk, oil and eggs. Stir into the flour mixture.

Divide the batter among the muffin cups. Bake for 20 minutes, or until a wooden cocktail stick inserted in the centre of a cupcake comes out clean.

To make the icing: In a small bowl, combine the cream cheese, sweetener, green tea and cardamom. Mix well. Spread over the tops of the cooled cupcakes.

PER CUPCAKE: 322 calories, 12g protein, 13g carbohydrates, 27g total fat, 6g saturated fat, 7g fibre, 320mg sodium

TART TANGERINE CUPCAKES

PREP TIME: 5 MINUTES | **TOTAL TIME:** 25 MINUTES + COOLING TIME

Makes 12 cupcakes

When in season, tangerines can be used to make a wonderfully flavourful, tart cupcake with the wheat-free baking mix. If tangerines are unavailable, you can make these orangey cupcakes with mandarin oranges (though 3 or 4 will be required) or navel oranges.

CUPCAKES

460g (1lb) All-Purpose Baking Mix (page 19)

Sweetener equivalent to 230g (8oz) sugar

½ tsp sea salt

225ml (8fl oz) tangerine juice or orange juice

3 eggs

ICING

230g (8oz) cream cheese, at room temperature

Sweetener equivalent to 115g (4oz) sugar

2 tsp tangerine juice or orange juice

Preheat the oven to 180°C/350°F/Gas mark 4. Place paper cases in a 12-cup muffin tin.

To make the cupcakes: In a large bowl, combine the baking mix, sweetener and salt. Mix well. In a cup, reserve 2 teaspoons of the juice for the icing. Add the remaining juice to the dry ingredients and stir well. Allow to stand for 1 to 2 minutes. Whisk the eggs and stir into the mixture.

Divide the batter among the muffin cups. Bake for 20 minutes, or until a wooden cocktail stick inserted in the centre of a cupcake comes out clean.

To make the icing: In a small bowl, combine the cream cheese, sweetener and the reserved 2 teaspoons juice. Mix well. Spread over the tops of the cooled cupcakes.

PER CUPCAKE: 303 calories, 11g protein, 13g carbohydrates, 25g total fat, 5g saturated fat, 6g fibre, 327mg sodium

MACADAMIA–SPICE MUFFINS

PREP TIME: 5 MINUTES | **TOTAL TIME:** 30 MINUTES

Makes 12 muffins

Macadamia nuts join cinnamon and nutmeg in this healthy and filling muffin. Remember: In this wheat-free lifestyle, unhealthy ingredients are eliminated – fat is *not* one of them. So enjoy your reacquaintance with high-fat macadamia nuts!

460g (1lb) All-Purpose Baking Mix
(page 19)

1½ tsp bicarbonate of soda

Sweetener equivalent to
345g (12oz) sugar

100g (3½oz) chopped macadamia nuts

1 tsp ground cinnamon

½ tsp ground nutmeg

½ tsp sea salt

1 tbsp lemon juice or vinegar

110ml (4fl oz) water

2 tbsp black treacle

3 eggs

Preheat the oven to 180°C/350°F/Gas mark 4. Grease a 12-cup muffin tin.

In a large bowl, combine the baking mix, bicarbonate of soda, sweetener, nuts, cinnamon, nutmeg and salt. Mix well.

In a small bowl, combine the lemon juice or vinegar, water and black treacle and mix. Add to the dry mixture and mix thoroughly.

In a small bowl, whisk the eggs. Add to the batter and mix thoroughly.

Divide the batter among the prepared muffin cups. Bake for 25 minutes, or until a wooden cocktail stick inserted in the centre of a muffin comes out clean.

PER MUFFIN: 299 calories, 11g protein, 14g carbohydrates, 25g total fat, 3g saturated fat, 7g fibre, 425mg sodium

APPLE STREUSEL MUFFINS

PREP TIME: 10 MINUTES | **TOTAL TIME:** 30 MINUTES

Makes 12 muffins

If you like coffee cake with crumbly streusel topping, here's a little nostalgia for you – with none of the heartache!

The streusel topping works with any sweetener, but xylitol works the best, as it creates the sturdiest and most crumbly end result.

460g (1lb) All-Purpose Baking Mix (page 19)

Sweetener equivalent to 115g (4oz) sugar

1 tsp ground cinnamon

¼ tsp ground nutmeg

½ tsp sea salt

270g (10oz) unsweetened apple purée

3 eggs

1 tbsp black treacle

125g (4½oz) butter, cut into small pieces

Preheat the oven to 160°C/325°F/Gas mark 3. Place paper cases in a 12-cup muffin tin.

In a large bowl, combine the baking mix, sweetener, cinnamon, nutmeg and salt. Mix well. Set aside a quarter of the mixture in a medium bowl. In a small bowl, combine the apple purée and eggs and stir until smooth. Add to the dry mixture and stir to combine. Divide the batter among the muffin cups.

To make the streusel topping, add the black treacle to the reserved dry mixture. Cut in the butter until the mixture becomes crumbly. Spoon gently over the tops of the muffins. Bake for 20 minutes, or until a wooden cocktail stick inserted in the centre of a muffin comes out clean.

PER MUFFIN: 311 calories, 10g protein, 14g carbohydrates, 27g total fat, 7g saturated fat, 7g fibre, 334mg sodium

APPLE PIE WHOOPIES

PREP TIME: 10 MINUTES | TOTAL TIME: 20 MINUTES + COOLING TIME

Makes 10 whoopies

As the name suggests, these little whoopies taste like a slice of apple pie. The kids will think it's dessert, but it's every bit as healthy as eating some nuts and apples!

CAKES

230g (8oz) All-Purpose Baking Mix (page 19)

90g (3oz) finely chopped walnuts

¼ tsp ground ginger or ground cardamom

Sweetener equivalent to 115g (4oz) sugar

2 tsp lemon juice

270g (10oz) unsweetened chunky apple purée

1 egg, whisked

GLAZE

2 tbsp xylitol

50g (2oz) cream cheese

½ tsp lemon juice

Preheat the oven to 180°C/350°F/Gas mark 4. Grease 10 cups of a whoopie baking tin.*

To make the cakes: In a large bowl, combine the baking mix, walnuts, ginger or cardamom and sweetener. Mix in the lemon juice, apple purée and egg until thoroughly combined.

Divide the batter among the whoopie cups. Bake for 10 minutes, or until slightly firm and golden. Allow to cool in the pan for 5 minutes. Invert onto a rack to cool completely.

To make the glaze: Meanwhile, in a small microwaveable bowl, combine the xylitol and cream cheese. Microwave on high power in 10-second increments until melted. Mix thoroughly. Add the lemon juice and stir to combine.

When the cakes have cooled, drizzle them with the glaze.

PER WHOOPIE: 218 calories, 7g protein, 9g carbohydrates, 19g total fat, 3g saturated fat, 5g fibre, 135mg sodium

*Note: Baking your wheat-free dough in the shallow cups of a whoopie tin provides easy and consistent baked final products. If you don't have a whoopie tin, these pies are easy to form with your hands. Just divide the dough into 50g (2oz) portions, then create 8cm (3in) patties and bake on a baking sheet lined with parchment paper.

CINNAMON ROLL WHOOPIES

PREP TIME: 10 MINUTES | **TOTAL TIME:** 20 MINUTES + COOLING TIME

Makes 10 whoopies

To make these whoopies seem even more like cinnamon rolls, you can add 30g (1¼oz) chopped pecans or chopped walnuts to the batter, or sprinkle the nuts on top of the glaze.

Serve these Cinnamon Roll Whoopies hot, topped with either the glaze or a pat of butter.

CAKES

230g (8oz) All-Purpose Baking Mix (page 19)

2 tsp ground cinnamon

Sweetener equivalent to 115g (4oz) sugar

1 tsp vanilla extract

110ml (4fl oz) double cream

2 tsp lemon juice

1 egg, whisked

GLAZE

2 tbsp xylitol

50g (2oz) cream cheese

½ tsp lemon juice

Preheat the oven to 180°C/350°F/Gas mark 4. Grease 10 cups of a whoopie baking tin.*

To make the cakes: In a large bowl, combine the baking mix, cinnamon and sweetener. Mix in the vanilla, cream, lemon juice and egg until thoroughly combined.

Divide the batter among the whoopie cups. Bake for 10 minutes, or until slightly firm and golden. Allow to cool in the pan for 5 minutes before inverting onto a rack.

To make the glaze: Meanwhile, in a small microwaveable bowl, combine the xylitol and cream cheese. Microwave on high power in 10-second increments until melted. Mix thoroughly. Add the lemon juice and stir to combine.

Drizzle the cakes with the glaze.

PER WHOOPIE: 188 calories, 6g protein, 7g carbohydrates, 16g total fat, 4g saturated fat, 4g fibre, 130mg sodium

* See note on opposite page.

PLUM JAM WHOOPIES

PREP TIME: 10 MINUTES | **TOTAL TIME:** 25 MINUTES + COOLING TIME

Makes 10 whoopies

Think of this recipe whenever you've made a batch of Plum–Chia Jam. It's a great way to make use of the leftovers!

CAKES

230g (8oz) All-Purpose Baking Mix (page 19)

Sweetener equivalent to 115g (4oz) sugar

115g (4oz) Plum–Chia Jam (page 51)

50ml (2fl oz) water

1 tsp lemon juice

1 egg, whisked

GLAZE

2 tbsp xylitol

50g (2oz) cream cheese

½ tsp lemon juice

Preheat the oven to 180°C/350°F/Gas mark 4. Grease 10 cups of a whoopie baking tin.*

To make the cakes: In a large bowl, combine the baking mix and sweetener. Mix in half of the jam, the water, lemon juice and egg until thoroughly combined.

Divide the batter among the 10 whoopie cups. Bake for 15 minutes, or until slightly firm and golden. Allow to cool in the pan for 5 minutes. Invert onto a rack to cool completely.

To make the glaze: Meanwhile, in a small microwaveable bowl, combine the xylitol and cream cheese. Microwave on high power in 10-second increments until melted. Mix thoroughly. Add the lemon juice and stir to combine.

Drizzle the cakes with the glaze. Spoon a small dollop of the remaining 2 tablespoons of jam on top of the glaze.

PER WHOOPIE: 167 calories, 6g protein, 9g carbohydrates, 13g total fat, 2g saturated fat, 4g fibre, 135mg sodium

* See note on page 204.

BERRY FOOL

PREP TIME: 5 MINUTES | **TOTAL TIME:** 5 MINUTES

Makes 4 servings

Three simple ingredients combine for a delicious treat that comes together in minutes.

150g (5oz) fresh berries of choice

Sweetener equivalent to
  2 tbsp sugar

225ml (8fl oz) double cream

In a food processor, pulse the berries with the sweetener until crushed, about 10 pulses. In a large bowl, with an electric mixer on high speed, beat the cream until stiff peaks form. Gently fold in the berries. Spoon into serving glasses and serve immediately or chill to serve later.

PER SERVING: 223 calories, 2g protein, 5g carbohydrates, 22g total fat, 14g saturated fat, 2g fibre, 23mg sodium

MOCHA KEFIRS

PREP TIME: 1 MINUTE | **TOTAL TIME:** 2 MINUTES

Makes 2 servings

If you haven't had kefir, a fermented milk drink, you are in for a real treat. This is like eating melted ice cream!

500g (18oz) kefir or whole milk yoghurt

Sweetener equivalent to
55g (2oz) sugar

1 tsp instant coffee granules

1 tbsp unsweetened
cocoa powder

In a blender, combine the kefir, sweetener, coffee granules and cocoa. Blend at medium speed until thick.

PER SERVING: 120 calories, 11g protein, 14g carbohydrates, 2g total fat, 1g saturated fat, 1g fibre, 123mg sodium

STRAWBERRY KEFIRS

PREP TIME: 1 MINUTE | **TOTAL TIME:** 2 MINUTES

Makes 2 servings

This kefir is a hit with kids. It can easily be altered to create blueberry, blackberry or mixed berry kefirs too.

500g (18oz) kefir or whole milk yoghurt

Sweetener equivalent to 55g (2oz) sugar

75g (3oz) fresh or frozen strawberries

2 mint sprigs, for garnish (optional)

In a blender, combine the kefir, sweetener and strawberries. Blend at medium speed until thick.

Serve as is or garnished with mint sprigs, if desired.

PER SERVING: 122 calories, 11g protein, 15g carbohydrates, 2g total fat, 1g saturated fat, 1g fibre, 124mg sodium

LEMON MOUSSE

PREP TIME: 5 MINUTES | **TOTAL TIME:** 15 MINUTES

Makes 6 servings

This quick, light dessert takes only 15 minutes to whip up but yields a wonderfully thick, rich mousse. I like serving it topped with fresh raspberries.

225ml (8fl oz) double cream

110g (4oz) cream cheese,
   at room temperature

Grated zest and juice of 1 lemon

Sweetener equivalent to 1 tbsp sugar

1 tsp vanilla extract

In a large bowl, with an electric mixer on high speed, beat the cream until stiff peaks form. Set aside.

In a separate bowl, with the same mixer at medium speed, beat the cream cheese, lemon zest and juice, sweetener and vanilla until blended. Gently fold the reserved whipped cream into the cream cheese mixture until thoroughly combined. Serve immediately or chill to serve later.

PER SERVING: 199 calories, 2g protein, 3g carbohydrates, 20g total fat, 12g saturated fat, 0g fibre, 75mg sodium

VANILLA CUSTARD

PREP TIME: 5 MINUTES | **TOTAL TIME:** 15 MINUTES + CHILLING TIME

Makes 4 servings

In the age of processed foods, many people have forgotten the simple art of making custard. Here is the basic recipe that can serve as the basis for a wide variety of rich custards, just by adding fresh or frozen berries, some unsweetened cocoa powder and dark chocolate chips or chopped nuts. (You can also take the finished, cooled custard and process it in an ice cream maker according to the manufacturer's directions. Also note that the addition of the custard step allows the use of coconut milk in place of dairy cream while maintaining a thick texture and smooth mouthfeel, a perennial struggle with dairy-free ice custards.)

350ml (12fl oz) double cream or tinned coconut milk

4 egg yolks

Sweetener equivalent to 115g (4oz) sugar

¼ tsp sea salt

1 tsp vanilla extract

1 tbsp butter, at room temperature

In a medium saucepan over a medium-high heat, heat the cream or coconut milk for 5 minutes, stirring with a wooden spoon, or just until bubbles start to form around the edges. Meanwhile, in a medium bowl, whisk together the egg yolks, sweetener, salt and vanilla. Gradually whisk the hot cream or coconut milk into the yolk mixture until blended.

Pour back into the saucepan. Cook over a medium heat for 5 minutes, stirring constantly, or until the mixture thickens. Remove from the heat and whisk in the butter until thoroughly incorporated and the custard is smooth.

Pour into a clean bowl and place clingfilm directly on the surface to prevent a skin from forming. Chill until ready to serve.

PER SERVING: 394 calories, 5g protein, 3g carbohydrates, 41g total fat, 24g saturated fat, 0g fibre, 166mg sodium

CARAMEL SAUCE

PREP TIME: 5 MINUTES | **TOTAL TIME:** 15 MINUTES

Makes 145ml (5fl oz)

This recipe is similar to the Vanilla Glaze (page 215), just cooked a bit longer to create the deep flavour and golden brown colour of caramel. Serve this caramel sauce on top of Vanilla Custard (page 211), drizzled on Cinnamon Doughnuts (page 196) or over Apple Streusel Muffins (page 203).

60g (2½oz) butter

35g (1¼oz) xylitol

50ml (2fl oz) double cream

½ tsp vanilla extract

In a small saucepan over a medium-high heat, combine the butter and xylitol. Mix well, then stop stirring as it heats. Allow the butter to brown and the xylitol to melt, occasionally gently swirling the saucepan, for 5 minutes.

Remove the saucepan from the heat. In a measuring cup or small bowl, combine the cream and vanilla. Stir, 1 tablespoon at a time, into the butter mixture. Be careful, as the mixture will bubble up and may spurt. Continue adding the cream mixture and stirring until incorporated. Allow the sauce to cool for 5 minutes before serving.

PER 1 TBSP: 53 calories, 0g protein, 1g carbohydrates, 6g total fat, 3g saturated fat, 0g fibre, 6mg sodium

LEMON WHIPPED CREAM

PREP TIME: 5 MINUTES | **TOTAL TIME:** 5 MINUTES

Makes 260ml (9fl oz)

Serve this flavourful cream with a few berries for a last-minute delicious dessert.

225ml (8fl oz) double cream

1 tsp grated lemon zest

1 tbsp lemon juice

In a large bowl, with an electric mixer on high speed, beat the cream until stiff peaks form. Gently stir in the lemon zest and juice. Use immediately or chill, covered, for up to 1 day.

PER 1 TBSP: 35 calories, 0g protein, 0g carbohydrates, 4g total fat, 2g saturated fat, 0g fibre, 4mg sodium

CHOCOLATE GLAZE

PREP TIME: 5 MINUTES | **TOTAL TIME:** 10 MINUTES + COOLING TIME

Makes 340g (12oz)

Drizzle this glaze over biscuits, cookies, cupcakes or muffins. For a dairy-free version, substitute coconut milk for the cream. Increase or decrease the quantity of cream to thin or thicken the glaze.

2 bars (100g/3½oz each) dark chocolate (85% cocoa), chopped

2 tbsp butter, softened

110ml (4fl oz) double cream

In the top of a double boiler, place the chocolate over simmering water and stir until melted. Remove from the heat and stir in the butter until melted. Stir in the cream until smooth and well combined. Allow to cool for several minutes before dipping or coating.

PER 1 TBSP: 80 calories, 1g protein, 5g carbohydrates, 8g total fat, 4g saturated fat, 1g fibre, 12mg sodium

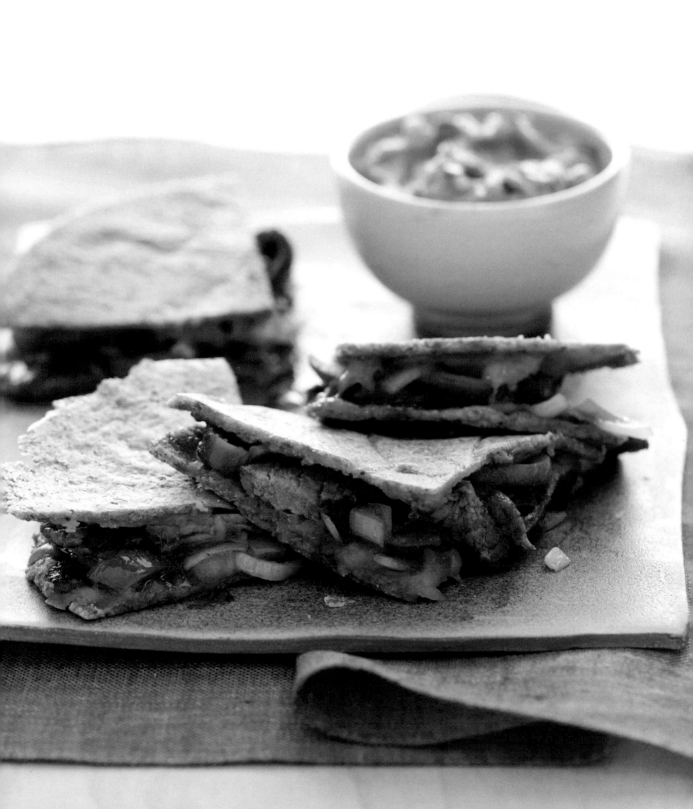

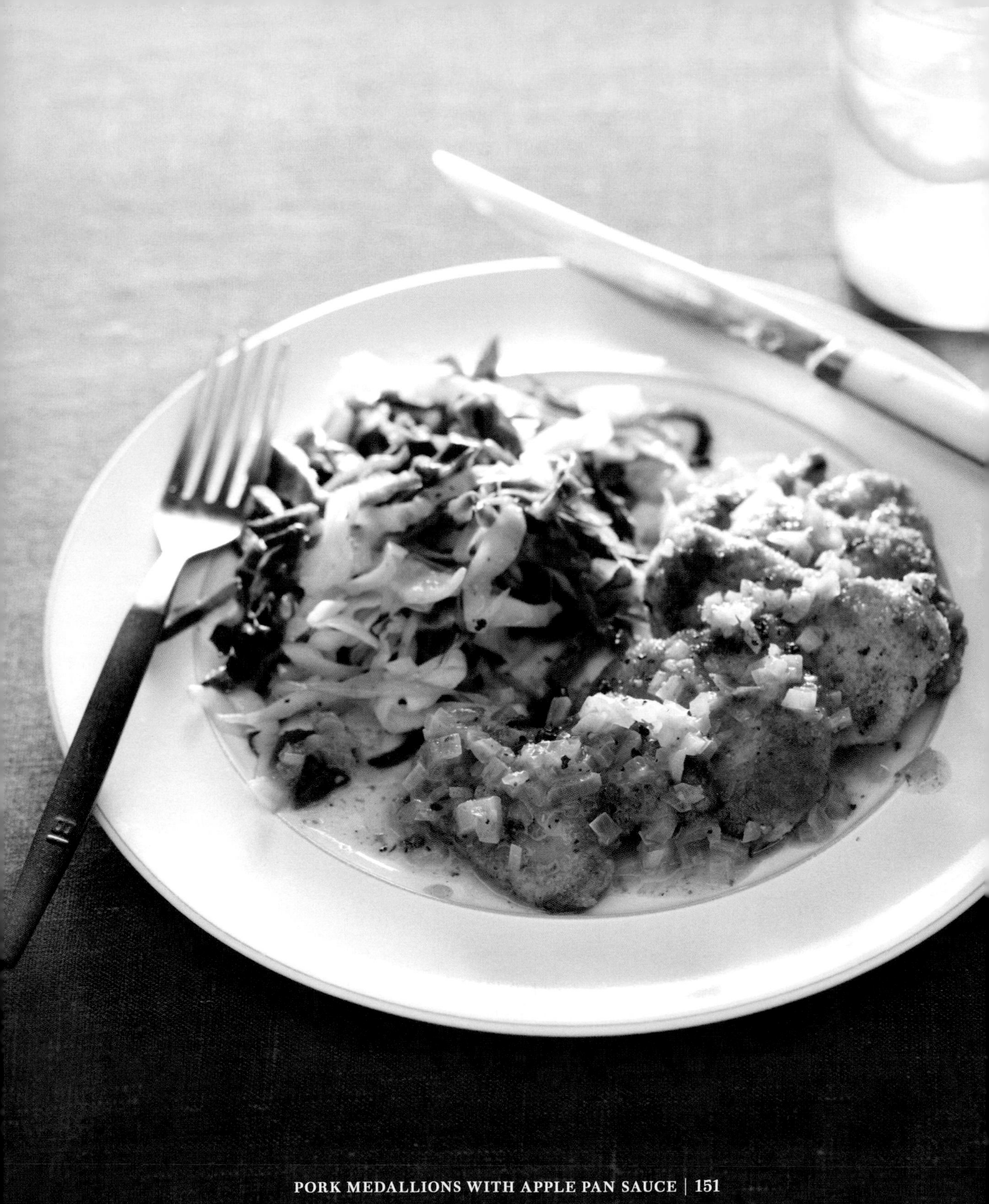

MOROCCAN CHICKEN WITH ROASTED PEPPERS | 156

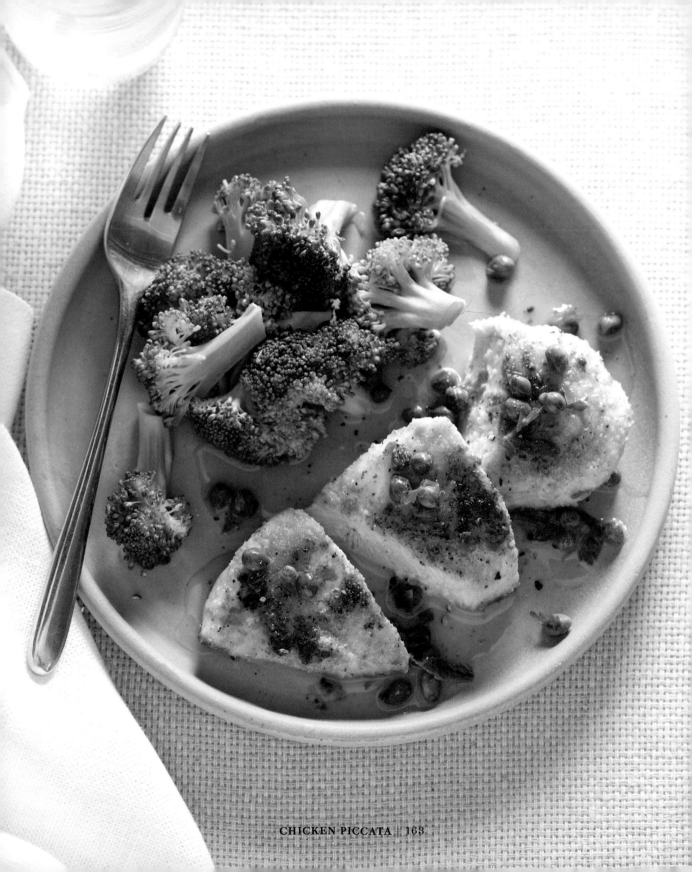

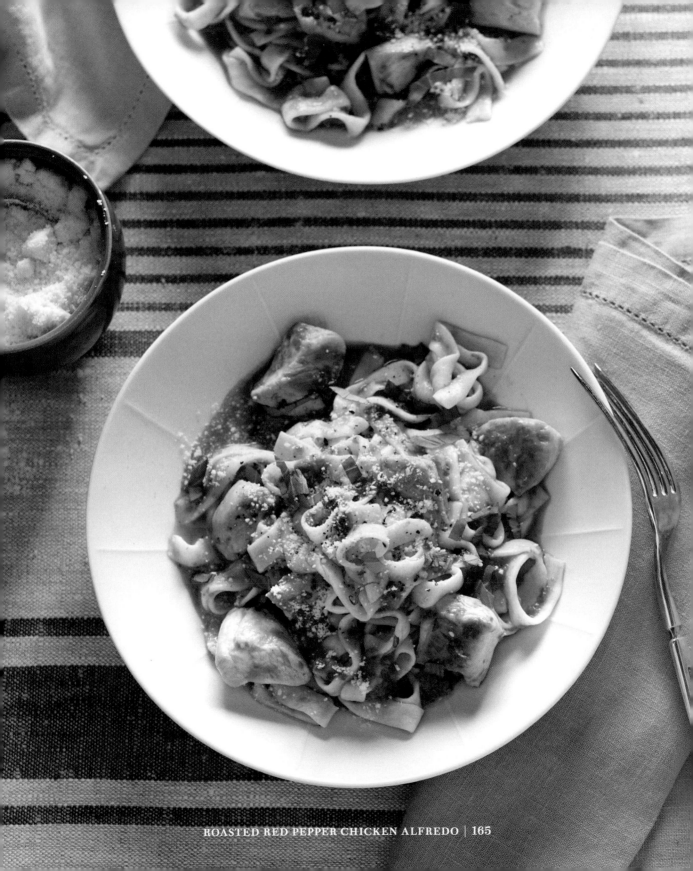

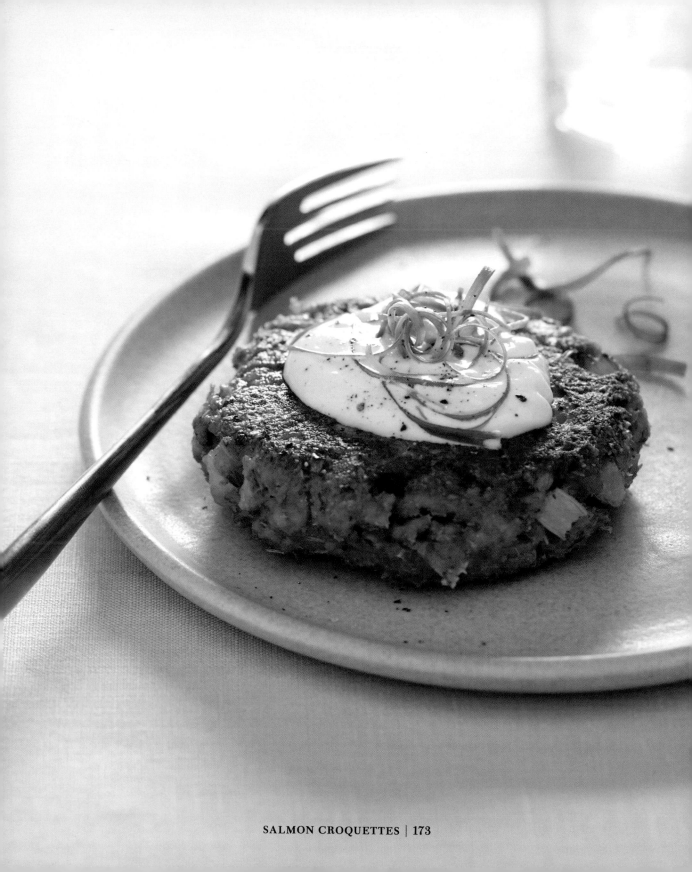

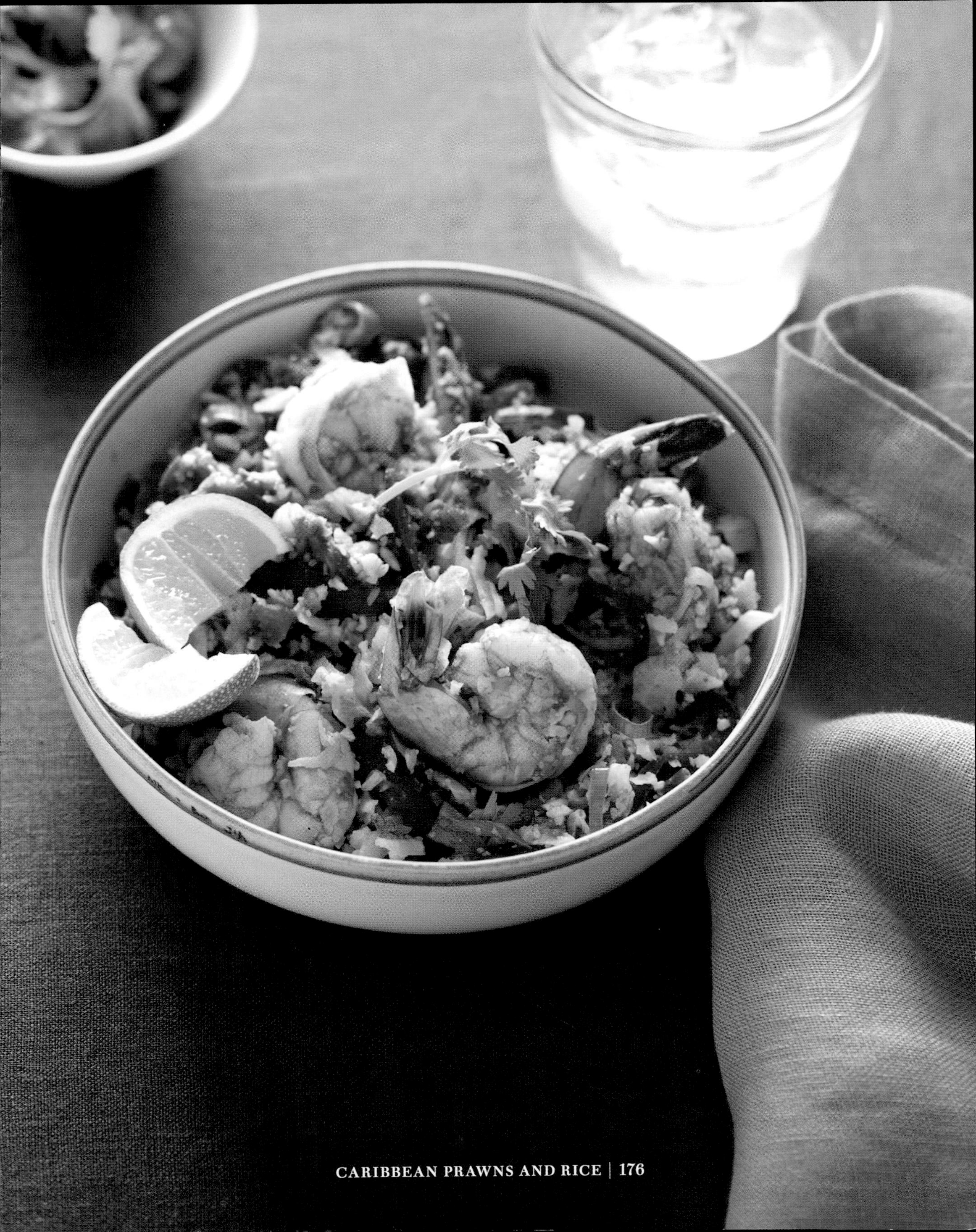

CARIBBEAN PRAWNS AND RICE |

KALE, ONION AND GOAT'S CHEESE PIZZA | 185

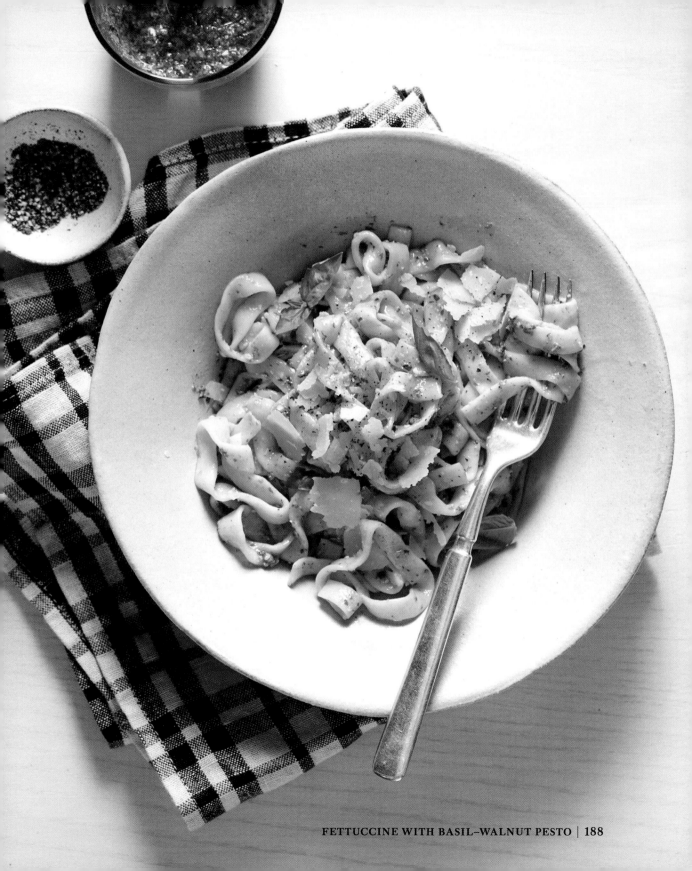

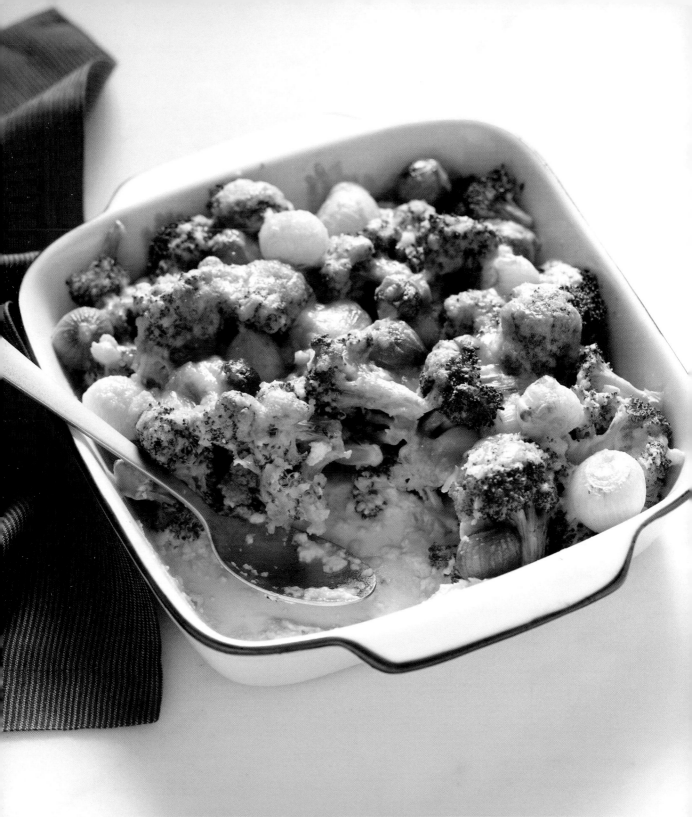

COCONUT–CHOCOLATE TART | 194

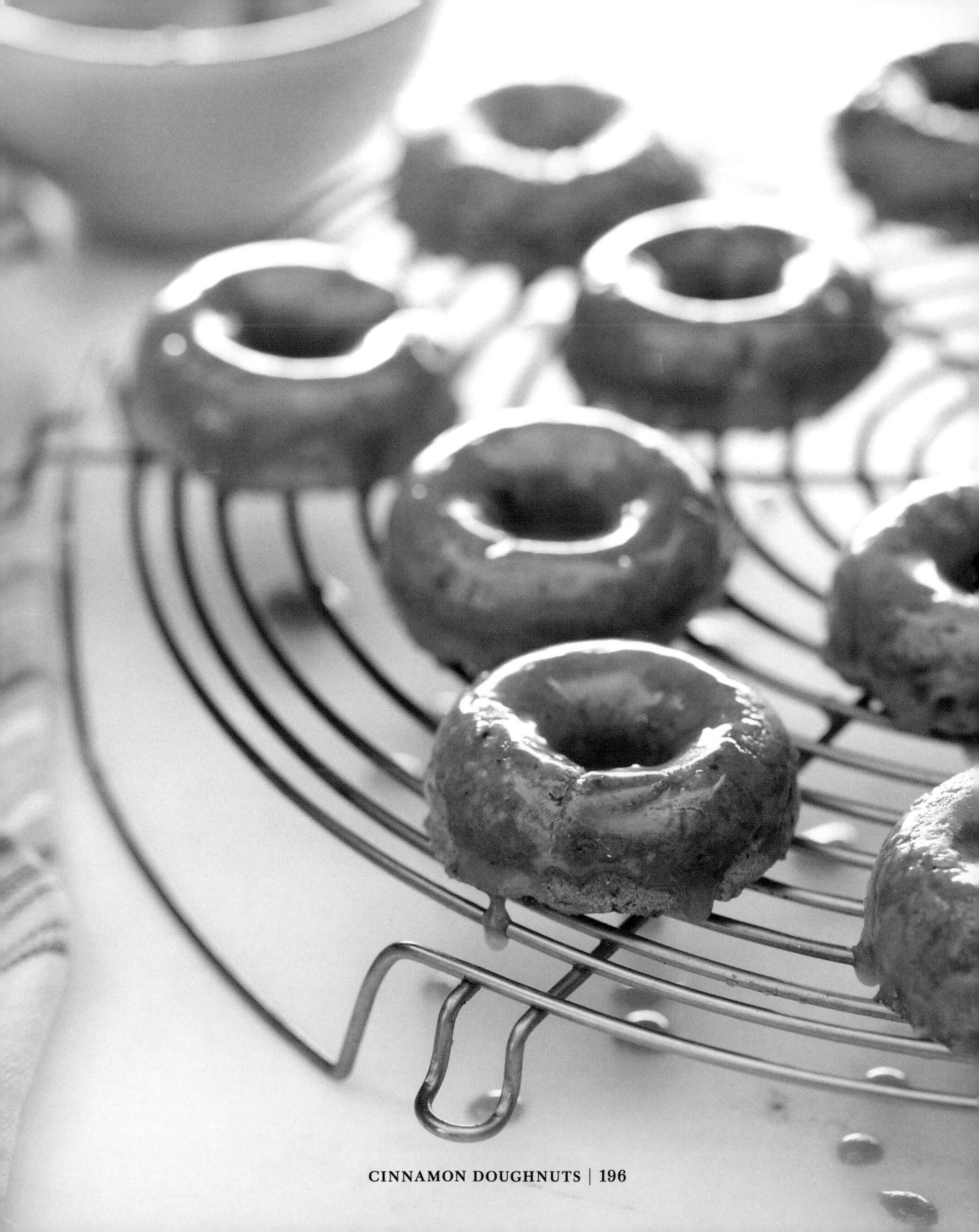

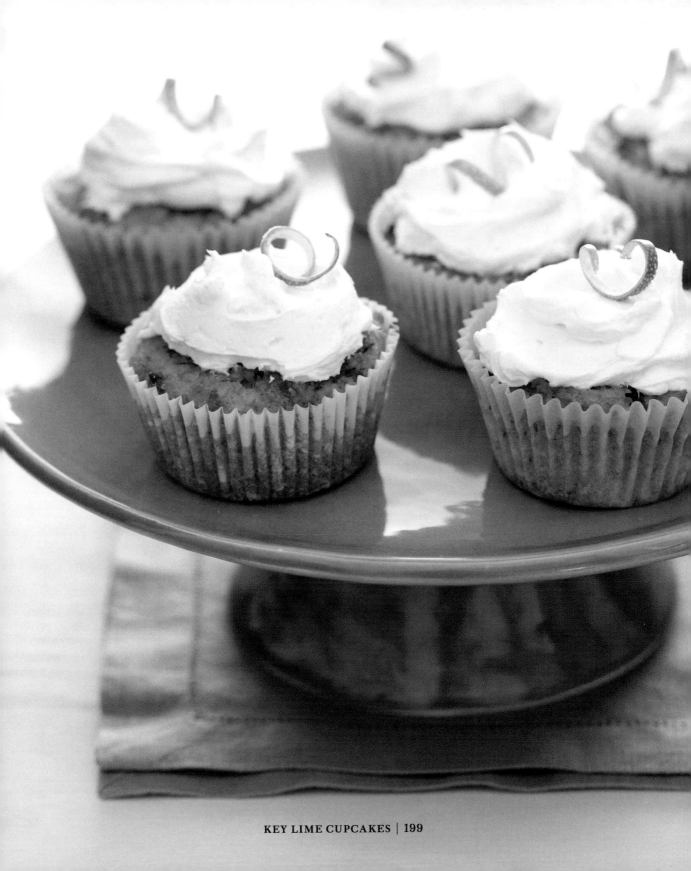

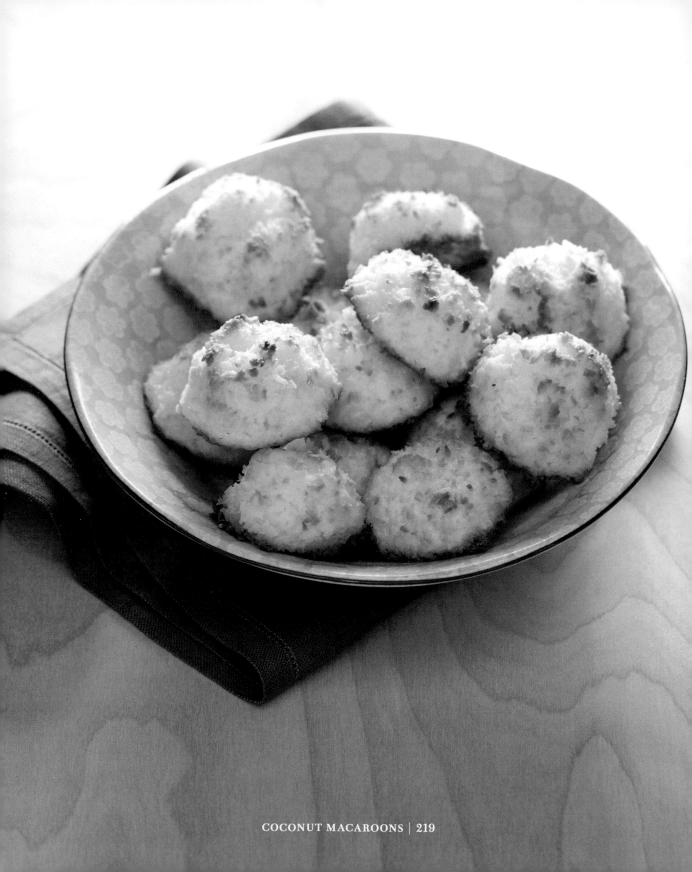

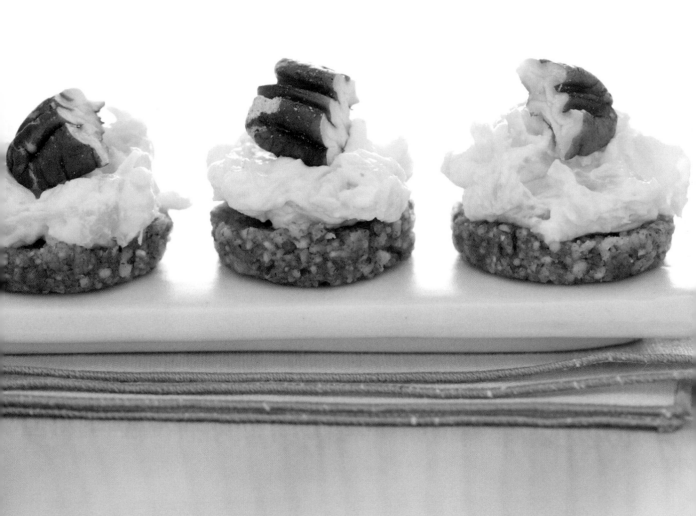

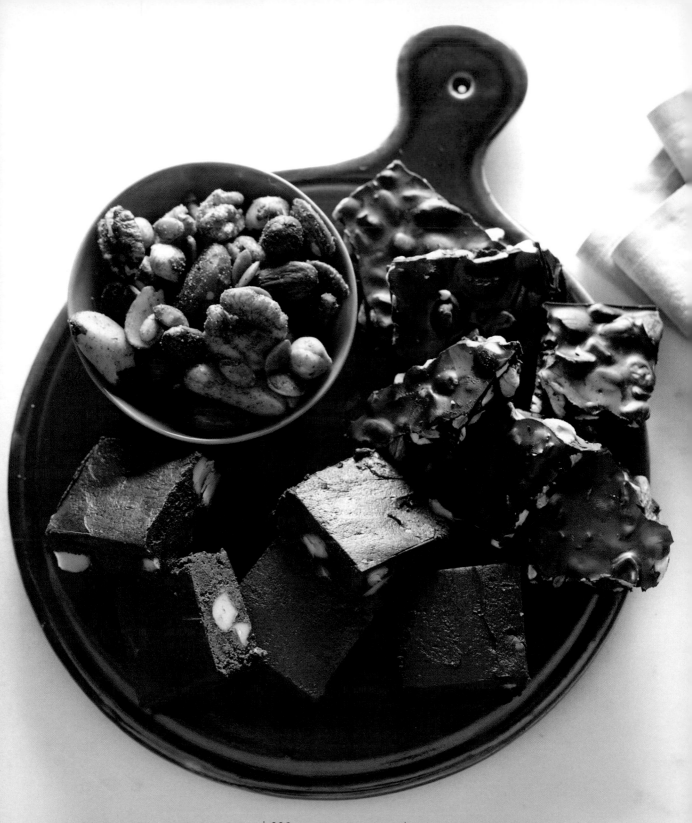

VANILLA GLAZE

PREP TIME: 5 MINUTES | **TOTAL TIME:** 5 MINUTES + COOLING TIME

Makes 90g (3oz)

This glaze achieves a caramel-like texture due to the unique properties of xylitol, the sugar replacement that most behaves like sugar in baking.

50ml (2fl oz) double cream

½ tsp vanilla extract

25g (1oz) xylitol

1 tbsp butter

In a small saucepan over a low heat, heat the cream, vanilla and xylitol until frothy, stirring constantly. Cook for 1 to 2 minutes, stirring constantly, or until bubbles form around the side of the saucepan. Do not scorch. Remove from the heat. Stir in the butter until smooth. Allow to cool to achieve the desired thickness before drizzling, dipping or coating.

PER 1 TBSP: 20 calories, 0g protein, 0g carbohydrates, 2g total fat, 1g saturated fat, 0g fibre, 8mg sodium

STRAWBERRY GLAZE

PREP TIME: 5 MINUTES | **TOTAL TIME:** 15 MINUTES + COOLING TIME

Makes 400g (14oz)

This simple glaze makes a syrupy topping for ice cream or custard, pancakes or Breakfast Cheesecake (page 74).

Note that xylitol was chosen as the sweetener in this recipe because of its unique glazing properties. Other sweeteners, such as stevia and erythritol, should not be substituted, as they will not yield the glaze effect.

600g (1lb 5oz) fresh strawberries, hulled and quartered

4 tbsp xylitol

In a food chopper, food processor or blender, pulse the strawberries and xylitol until puréed.

In a medium saucepan over a medium heat, heat the strawberry mixture. Allow to bubble and froth. Reduce the heat to low.

Cook for 5 minutes, stirring frequently, or until the mixture thickens and becomes syrupy. Be careful not to let the mixture boil or burn. Remove from the heat and allow to cool.

PER 1 TBSP: 8 calories, 0g protein, 2g carbohydrates, 0g total fat, 0g saturated fat, 0g fibre, 0mg sodium

CHOCOLATE ICING

PREP TIME: 5 MINUTES | **TOTAL TIME:** 5 MINUTES

Makes 295g (10½oz)

Here's a rich, buttery icing as good as or better than anything ready-made. Save a small batch in the refrigerator to put on top of your Coconut–Chocolate Quick Muffin (page 87) for breakfast.

125g (4½oz) butter, at room temperature

115g (4oz) cream cheese, at room temperature

Sweetener equivalent to 115g (4oz) sugar

30g (1¼oz) unsweetened cocoa powder

1 tbsp double cream

1 tsp vanilla extract

In a medium bowl, with an electric mixer on medium speed, cream the butter, cream cheese and sweetener until fluffy. Blend in the cocoa, cream and vanilla and beat until smooth.

PER 1 TBSP: 66 calories, 1g protein, 1g carbohydrates, 7g total fat, 4g saturated fat, 0g fibre, 59mg sodium

VANILLA ICING

PREP TIME: 5 MINUTES | **TOTAL TIME:** 5 MINUTES

Makes 260g (9oz)

This quick vanilla icing works on desserts such as cakes and muffins as well as an Apple–Spice Quick Muffin for breakfast (page 85).

115g (4oz) butter, at room temperature

115g (4oz) cream cheese, at room temperature

Sweetener equivalent to 115g (4oz) sugar

1 tbsp double cream

1 tsp vanilla extract

In a medium bowl, with an electric mixer on medium speed, cream the butter, cream cheese and sweetener until fluffy. Blend in the cream and vanilla and beat until smooth.

PER 1 TBSP: 77 calories, 1g protein, 1g carbohydrates, 8g total fat, 5g saturated fat, 0g fibre, 58mg sodium

COCONUT MACAROONS

PREP TIME: 10 MINUTES | **TOTAL TIME:** 25 MINUTES

Makes 8 macaroons

These simple coconut macaroons require just a few ingredients but will be sure to delight! As with all of the snacks and desserts in this book, because all unhealthy ingredients have been removed and are replaced with healthy substitutes, you can have these macaroons for breakfast as well as for dessert.

To make Orange–Clove–Coconut Macaroons, after adding the sweetener to the egg white mixture, fold in ¼ teaspoon ground cloves, the grated zest of 1 orange and the juice of half an orange.

3 egg whites

¼ tsp cream of tartar

120g (4oz) shredded or desiccated
    unsweetened coconut

Sweetener equivalent to
    115g (4oz) sugar*

Preheat the oven to 180°C/350°F/Gas mark 4. Line a baking sheet with parchment paper.

In a large bowl, with an electric mixer on high speed, beat the egg whites and cream of tartar until stiff peaks form.

Fold the coconut and sweetener into the egg white mixture.

Scoop the mixture onto the baking sheet to form 8 mounds. Bake for 15 minutes, or until golden and slightly firm to the touch. Allow to cool before serving.

PER MACAROON: 167 calories, 3g protein, 5g carbohydrates, 15g total fat, 13g saturated fat, 3g fibre, 27mg sodium

*Note: If using a sweetener with large granules, such as xylitol, grind it in a food processor for 30 seconds, to reduce it to a finer powder, before proceeding with the recipe.

LEMON-PINEAPPLE SNOWBALLS

PREP TIME: 5 MINUTES | **TOTAL TIME:** 15 MINUTES + CHILLING TIME

Makes 30 snowballs

This may be the fastest way to keep the kids happy in their wheat-free lifestyle: only 15 minutes!

The zesty tropical combination of lemon and pineapple brings these little balls of goodness to life.

135g (5oz) shredded or desiccated unsweetened coconut, divided

1 tin (230g/8oz) crushed pineapple, drained

Grated zest and juice from 1 lemon

225g (8oz) cream cheese, at room temperature

Sweetener equivalent to 3 tbsp sugar

In a food chopper or food processor, briefly pulse 120g (4oz) of the coconut to reduce the size of the coconut shreds. Pour into a large bowl. Place the remaining coconut in a shallow bowl or pie plate and set aside.

To the bowl, add the pineapple, lemon zest and juice, cream cheese and sweetener. Mix thoroughly.

Use a tablespoon to scoop the mixture into small mounds onto a plate or baking sheet, and then roll into 2–3cm (1in) balls. If the mixture sticks to your hands, moisten them with water. Roll balls in the reserved coconut, return to the plate or baking sheet, and chill for at least 30 minutes before serving.

PER SNOWBALL: 77 calories, 1g protein, 3g carbohydrates, 7g total fat, 5g saturated fat, 1g fibre, 26mg sodium

PECAN-PINEAPPLE BITES

PREP TIME: 15 MINUTES | **TOTAL TIME:** 15 MINUTES + CHILLING TIME

Makes 30 bites

These itsy-bitsy bite-sized 'bites' are deceptively filling. They are fun and cute enough for the kids, but elegant enough to serve to company.

125g (4½oz) ground pecans

45g (1½oz) butter, melted

Sweetener equivalent to 55g (2oz) sugar

1 tin (230g/8oz) crushed pineapple, drained

225g (8oz) cream cheese, at room temperature

30 pecan halves

On a baking sheet or large plate, arrange 30 mini paper cases.

In a medium bowl, combine the ground pecans, butter and sweetener. Mix thoroughly. Spoon evenly into the cases, pressing down with your fingers or a spoon. Set aside.

In another bowl, combine the pineapple and cream cheese. Stir until well blended.

Spoon evenly over the pecan cases. Place 1 pecan half on top of each. Chill for at least 30 minutes.

PER BITE: 77 calories, 1g protein, 2g carbohydrates, 8g total fat, 2.5g saturated fat, 1g fibre, 34mg sodium

COGNAC TRUFFLES

PREP TIME: 5 MINUTES | **TOTAL TIME:** 30 MINUTES

Makes 30 truffles

Cognac is a deliciously wheat-free and indulgent liquor that mixes perfectly with cocoa. This simple recipe yields a creamy, melt-in-your-mouth treat that lingers with the flavours of your favourite cognac. Serve with espresso at the end of an elegant dinner.

170g (6oz) plain (85% cocoa) chocolate, chopped

1 tbsp black treacle

Sweetener equivalent to 115g (4oz) sugar

2 tbsp cognac

175ml (6fl oz) double cream

30g (1¼oz) unsweetened cocoa powder

Line a baking sheet or large plate with parchment paper.

In the top of a double boiler, place the chocolate over simmering water and stir until melted. Stir in the black treacle, sweetener and cognac. Remove from the heat.

Meanwhile, in a large bowl, with an electric mixer on high speed, beat the cream until stiff peaks form. Fold into the chocolate mixture until all the cream is incorporated. The mixture will be relatively stiff.

Place the cocoa powder in a small bowl. Use a tablespoon to scoop out the truffle mixture and, using your hands, form it into balls. Set on the baking sheet or plate. Roll the balls in the cocoa to coat. Chill in an airtight container for up to 1 week.

PER TRUFFLE: 54 calories, 1g protein, 3g carbohydrates, 5g total fat, 3g saturated fat, 1g fibre, 4mg sodium

MACADAMIA NUT FUDGE

PREP TIME: 5 MINUTES | **TOTAL TIME:** 15 MINUTES + CHILLING TIME

Makes 32 servings

You will be hard-pressed to find anything more indulgent than fudge. Yet here it is in a cookbook designed for health! The macadamias can be replaced with your choice of nuts, such as walnuts, pecans or pistachios.

225g (8oz) plain (85% cocoa) chocolate, chopped

225g (8oz) cream cheese, at room temperature

Sweetener equivalent to 230g (8oz) sugar

6 tbsp double cream

1 tsp vanilla extract

1 tsp almond extract

120g (4oz) unsalted dry-roasted macadamia nuts, chopped

Grease a 20 x 20cm (8 x 8in) baking dish or baking tin.

In the top of a double boiler, place the chocolate over simmering water and stir until melted. Alternatively, place the chocolate in a microwaveable bowl and microwave on high power in 15-second increments, stirring in between, until smooth.

Meanwhile, in a medium bowl, with an electric mixer on medium speed, beat the cream cheese and sweetener until creamy. Add the cream, vanilla and almond extract and mix to combine. Stir in the chocolate until well combined. Stir in the nuts. Spread into the baking dish or baking tin and chill until firm.

PER SERVING: 92 calories, 2g protein, 3g carbohydrates, 10g total fat, 5g saturated fat, 1g fibre, 24mg sodium

DARK CHOCOLATE-NUT CRUNCH

PREP TIME: 5 MINUTES | **TOTAL TIME:** 10 MINUTES + CHILLING TIME

Makes 15 servings

This rich treat is great as is or spread with a bit of almond butter.

225g (8oz) plain (85% cocoa) chocolate, chopped

1 tsp coconut oil

280g (10oz) mixed raw or dry-roasted nuts (such as pistachios, cashews, almonds, Brazil nuts, walnuts, pecans and macadamia nuts), roughly chopped

Line a 23 x 23cm (9 x 9in) baking dish with parchment paper or foil.

In the top of a double boiler, place the chocolate and oil over simmering water and stir until smooth. Remove from the heat. Add the nuts, stirring to coat with the chocolate.

Spread the mixture evenly into the baking dish. Refrigerate for 30 minutes, or until set. Break into pieces.

PER SERVING: 170 calories, 5g protein, 8g carbohydrates, 16g total fat, 6g saturated fat, 4g fibre, 87mg sodium

SPICY MIXED NUTS

PREP TIME: 5 MINUTES | **TOTAL TIME:** 15 MINUTES

Makes 620g (1lb 6oz)

Mixed nuts purchased at the shops are invariably coated with hydrogenated ('trans') fats to allow the salt to stick to the nuts. This converts something wonderful for health – nuts – into something awful for health due to the trans fats. Tasty dry-roasted nuts without the nastiness of trans fats can be re-created very easily.

For simplicity and time, I put the seasoning mixes to work. However, if desired, they are easily substituted with your choice of seasonings, such as garlic powder, onion powder, paprika, ground pepper and salt.

560g (1lb 3oz) mixed raw nuts (such as almonds, walnuts, pecans, pistachios, Brazil nuts and hazelnuts; also consider raw pumpkin seeds or sunflower seeds)

2 tbsp coconut oil, melted

1–2 tbsp Cajun Seasoning Mix (page 58) or Taco Seasoning Mix (page 57)

½ tsp sea salt

Preheat the oven to 180°C/350°F/Gas mark 4.

In a large bowl, combine the nuts, oil, seasoning mix and salt. Toss until well mixed.

Spread on a shallow baking tin and bake for 10 minutes, stirring once, or until lightly toasted and fragrant.

PER 45G (1½OZ) SERVING: 193 calories, 5g protein, 6g carbohydrates, 18g total fat, 3g saturated fat, 3g fibre, 61mg sodium

CHOCOLATE PEANUT BUTTER CAKE

PREP TIME: 5 MINUTES | **TOTAL TIME:** 5 MINUTES

Makes 1 serving

Missing a sweet treat? This quick mini cake will satisfy any sweet tooth.

3 tbsp ground almonds/flour

1 tbsp ground golden flaxseeds

2 tbsp unsweetened
   cocoa powder

Sweetener equivalent to
   2 tbsp sugar

¼ tsp baking powder

¼ tsp salt

1 tbsp peanut butter, softened

2 tbsp milk

1 tbsp coconut oil or
   melted butter

In a coffee mug with a fork, stir together the ground almonds/flour, flaxseeds, cocoa powder, sweetener, baking powder and salt until smooth. Mix together the peanut butter, milk and oil or butter. Mix into the dry ingredients and microwave on high for 1 to 2 minutes until set. Eat with a dollop of Greek yoghurt or whipped cream.

PER SERVING: 313 calories, 9g protein, 15g carbohydrates, 29g total fat, 14g saturated fat, 8g fibre, 423mg sodium

MENUS FOR
SPECIAL OCCASIONS

HERE ARE THEMED menus to suit a number of special occasions, from Sunday Brunch to Pub Night to Chinese Takeaway. Of course, you can follow any of these menus even when it's not a special occasion, when you're just in the mood for an interesting meal!

Entire menus cannot, of course, be assembled in a 30-minute timeline, so plan accordingly. All menu items can be made from recipes in this cookbook except those marked with an asterisk (*).

FRIDAY NIGHT PIZZA

It's all about the pizza and the company you keep with Friday Night Pizza! There are endless variations on the combinations of meats, vegetables and cheeses for pizza; the two recipes provided in this cookbook are unique starting places. Since beer is a popular accompaniment to pizza, several safe beers are listed, too.

• Provolone, Prosciutto and Kalamata Olive Pizza (page 155) or Kale, Onion and Goat's Cheese Pizza (page 185)

• Apple Pie Whoopies (page 204) or Cinnamon Roll Whoopies (page 205) or Plum Jam Whoopies (page 206)

• Gluten-free beer or wheat-free but not gluten-free beer for the non-coeliac or non-gluten-sensitive

TEX-MEX NIGHT

Have some fresh salsa on hand for a fun and spicy Mexican Night!

- Guacamole (page 32) and Pitta Crisps (page 27)

- Barbecue Beef Quesadillas (page 140)

- Pepper and Beef Tortillas (page 145) or Chorizo–Prawn Tortillas (page 179)

- Taco Lettuce Wraps (page 144)

- Vanilla Custard (page 211) topped with crushed pecans, Chocolate Glaze (page 214) and cinnamon

PUB NIGHT

Get your family together for an evening of fun foods. Good news: although the menu sounds like a list of junk foods, none are junk!

These recipes transform ordinarily indulgent foods with unhealthy ingredients into healthy dishes with no downside. Enjoy your meal and don't be concerned about weight gain, heartburn or any of those nasty wheat-related worries!

- Spicy Mixed Nuts (page 227) or Chipotle Pepper Roasted Almonds (page 228)

- Barbecue Bacon-Wrapped Chicken (page 161)

- Spicy Chicken Thighs (page 157)

- Pepperoni Bread (page 108)

- Peanut Butter Cookies (page 221)

- Gluten-free beer or wheat-free but not gluten-free beer for the non-coeliac or non-gluten-sensitive

CHINESE TAKEAWAY

You won't be hungry in 2 hours after this Chinese meal! Be sure to have some gluten-free soy sauce or tamari on hand, if desired.

- Brewed green tea*

- Egg Drop Soup (page 95)

- Japanese Aubergine Stir-Fry over shirataki noodles (page 190)

- Pork Fried 'Rice' (page 133)

- Vanilla Custard (page 211) sprinkled with freshly ground or dried nutmeg or Pistachio–Green Tea Cupcakes (page 200)

SUMMER PICNIC

A refreshing salad, a light sandwich or wrap, cupcakes, sunlight . . . with no after-meal heartburn, sleepiness or weight gain: does life get any better than that?

- Cucumber, red onion and tomato salad* with Dilled Cucumber Yoghurt Sauce (page 38)

- Avocado–Ham Sandwiches (page 105) or Tex-Mex Egg Salad Wraps (page 113) or Pepperoni Pizza Wraps (page 116)

- Tart Tangerine Cupcakes (page 201)

ROMANTIC EVENING

Romantic dinners mean foods with subtle and fragrant nuances, not overly elaborate but prepared with care, ending with something lightly indulgent.

　　Wine and digestive suggestions are included for those so inclined.

- Moroccan Chicken with Roasted Peppers (page 156) or Parmesan-Crusted Cod (page 169) or Steak Béarnaise (page 136)

- Wines with dinner: Pinot Grigio with chicken or cod; Merlot or Cabernet Sauvignon with steak

- Artichokes, Pancetta and Kale with Shaved Parmesan (page 121) or Crab-Stuffed Mushrooms (page 127) or Italian Marinated Mushrooms (page 126)

- Tomato and Fennel Soup (page 94) or green salad with Moroccan Dressing (page 48)

- Cognac Truffles (page 224) or Double Chocolate Mini Cakes (page 198) or Coconut Macaroons (page 219)

- Courvoisier or other Cognac

FILM NIGHT

Here are finger foods to munch with your drama, love story or comedy!

- Spicy Mixed Nuts (page 227) or Horseradish–Soy Sauce Roasted Almonds (page 229)

- Dark Chocolate–Nut Crunch (page 226)

- Ice Cream Sandwiches (Vanilla Custard, page 211, sandwiched between two Peanut Butter Cookies, page 221) or Cinnamon Doughnuts (page 196)

ITALIAN NIGHT

Minus the Italian bread and wheat-based pasta, you can still have a wonderful and varied Italian-style meal that relies on the flavours of tomato, oregano, basil, mushrooms and red wine.

- Green salad with halved fresh mozzarella balls and cherry tomatoes,* topped with Spicy Italian Dressing (page 49)

- Italian Sausage Meatballs with Red Wine Sauce (page 109) served over shirataki fettuccine

- Italian Marinated Mushrooms (page 126) or Crab-Stuffed Mushrooms (page 127)

- Breakfast Cheesecake (page 74) with Strawberry Glaze (page 216)

NEW ORLEANS JAMBOREE

You don't need to wait for Fat Tuesday to enjoy the wonderful flavours of New Orleans! Finish this spicy dinner menu with the smooth coolness of vanilla custard topped with caramel, accompanied by a rich café au lait.

- Devilled eggs made with Spicy Cajun Mayo (page 42)

- Jambalaya (page 152) or Cajun Baked Fish with Prawn Cream Sauce (page 168) or Cajun Chicken Cutlets (page 162)

- Cajun Kale (page 124)

- Vanilla Custard (page 211) with pecans and Caramel Sauce (page 212)

- Café au lait*

INDIAN NIGHT

For an adventurous night of exotic foods, try this mix of flavourful Indian dishes, topped off with a burst of citrussy Lemon–Pineapple Snowballs and the heady flavours of chai tea.

If you are making more than one curried dish, consider distinguishing them by choosing different varieties of curry for each, such as vindaloo curry for the prawns and a garam masala mixture for the rice or vegetables.

- Curried 'Rice' (page 132) or Curried Vegetables (page 183)

- Indian Curry Prawns (page 180)

- Palak Paneer (page 186)

- Lemon–Pineapple Snowballs (page 222)

- Chai tea with coconut milk*

SUNDAY BRUNCH

This one will take some work! This is the sort of spread you might anticipate for a big family get-together. One interesting observation you may make: your guests will eat less than they would at a conventional Sunday brunch because your brunch contains no appetite stimulants. They can relish your wonderful cooking without worrying about gaining weight and – especially important for anyone with diabetes – without experiencing any substantial rise in blood sugar. You and your guests can just eat and enjoy it!

- Smoked Salmon Wraps (page 117)

- Wasabi Devilled Eggs (page 103)

- Cream of Mushroom Soup with Chives (page 92)

- Italian Sausage Meatballs with Red Wine Sauce (page 109)

- Crab-Stuffed Mushrooms (page 127) or Italian Marinated Mushrooms (page 126)

- Fillet of Fish Amandine (page 170)

- Chicken Piccata (page 163) or Barbecue Bacon-Wrapped Chicken (page 161)

- Roasted Courgette, Squash and Tomato Medley (page 131)

- Apple Streusel Muffins (page 203) or Key Lime Cupcakes (page 199) or Pistachio–Green Tea Cupcakes (page 200) or Tart Tangerine Cupcakes (page 201) or Macadamia–Spice Muffins (page 202)

- Optional: dry (brut or extra brut) Champagne, sparkling wine or prosecco

WINTER LUNCH

If you live in a colder climate like I do, you know how wonderful a hot lunch with familiar comfort foods can be on a cold winter day. Most conventional notions of comfort food, however, mean plenty of blood sugar problems and weight gain. As with all of my recipes, these comfort foods can be eaten . . . well, comfortably, without those sorts of worries!

- New England Clam Chowder (page 99) or Cream of Mushroom Soup with Chives (page 92)

- Balsamic Mushroom Wraps (page 115) or Tex-Mex Egg Salad Wraps (page 113)

- Berry–Coconut Mini Cheesecakes (page 195)

BACKYARD BARBECUE

Eating outdoors is one of the truly simple pleasures in life. In this menu, simplicity is the theme, allowing you to enjoy the sun and outdoors more with less cooking fuss. To simplify preparation, make the Pitta Crisps ahead of time or keep a supply on hand. Iced tea can likewise be made earlier in the day.

• Guacamole (page 32) and Pitta Crisps (page 27)

• Pork ribs* brushed with Barbecue Sauce (page 35)

• Grilled fresh asparagus or other vegetables*

• Coconut–Chocolate Tart (page 194)

• Iced tea with mint leaves*

APPENDIX
Wheat-Free Resources

THERE ARE PLENTY of resources available for people with coeliac disease or gluten sensitivity. They are primarily useful to help identify hidden sources of gluten, locate restaurants and shops that sell gluten-free foods, and find doctors familiar with the special needs of people who have coeliac disease.

Because *Wheat Belly* and the *Wheat Belly Cookbook* introduce the idea that wheat elimination is not just for people with coeliac disease or gluten sensitivity, but for everyone, the resources that target this larger audience are still limited, though they will probably grow rapidly as this concept catches on.

In the meantime, some resources for products, additional wheat-free recipes and more information are listed on the following pages. Resources for those who have coeliac disease or gluten sensitivity are included as well.

Nuts, Seeds, Ground Nuts and Flours

Sources for nuts, seeds, ground nuts and flours may be as close as your supermarket. However, it really pays to shop around, as prices vary widely (as much as sixfold – 600 per cent!). The most economical method is usually to grind nuts and flours yourself in a food chopper, food processor or coffee grinder. However, most major supermarkets and health food shops carry pre-ground nuts and flours. Ground seeds are rarely sold pre-ground but are very easy to grind from whole sesame, sunflower, chia or pumpkin seeds.

Bob's Red Mill is a brand that is available online and has an excellent source of high-quality (often organic) almond flour, coconut flour, chickpea flour and xanthan gum.

Trader Joe's is another affordable online source for nearly all the whole nuts and seeds you need. They also have ground almonds for a great price. Whole Foods Market is another, albeit high-cost, source for most nuts, seeds and flours.

The online retailers below have extensive choices of nuts, seeds, ground nuts and seeds and flours, including almonds, almond flour and chia.

www.nuts.com
www.ohnuts.com
www.nutstop.com
www.diamondnuts.com
www.nutsonthenet.com
www.nutiva.com

Sweeteners

Start with your supermarket or health food shop for liquid stevia, powdered stevia (pure stevia or made with inulin) or Truvía. Health food shops, in particular, typically have several choices of stevia, since it has been available for several years as a nutritional supplement.

Erythritol and xylitol are not always available in shops. Check health food shops, but you may need to order online. Nuts.com carries xylitol, and Amazon carries several brands of xylitol and erythritol, including NOW, KAL and Emerald Forest.

You can also find erythritol and xylitol at:

www.wheatfreemarket.com
www.luckyvitamin.com
www.4allvitamins.com
www.iherb.com

Monk Fruit (Luo han guo):

www.wheatfreemarket.com
www.intheraw.com

Shirataki Noodles

Bigger and better-stocked health food shops will often carry shirataki noodles, though look for them in the refrigerated section, not on the pasta shelf. If not available in your local shop, these noodles can be purchased online. Miracle and House Foods are two good brands.

Coeliac Disease Resources

Here are additional resources for individuals with coeliac disease or gluten sensitivity. They are useful for helping to identify foods containing gluten, and some of these organizations maintain lists of restaurants that accommodate safe gluten-free eating. The Gluten Intolerance Group, for instance, maintains a list of gluten-free restaurants searchable by state or zip code. The Celiac Disease Foundation's website also provides links to the websites of the various gluten-free food manufacturers. In the UK, Coeliac UK (www.coeliac.org.uk) provides a wealth of resources, as well as funding research into the disease.

These organizations also provide support to restaurants and food manufacturers needing guidance on creating a gluten-free food preparation environment. The National Foundation for Coeliac Awareness, for instance, offers a food service training programme.

These organizations are supported by donations and product sales. However, buyer beware: much of the revenue that supports these organizations comes from manufacturers of gluten-free foods. It means that they tend to steer you towards these products, which are best avoided entirely. Nonetheless, these organizations can serve as a useful starting place for more information relevant to coeliac disease and gluten sensitivity.

CeliacCorner
www.celiaccorner.com

Celiac Disease Foundation
www.celiac.org

Celiac Sprue Association
www.csaceliacs.info

Gluten Intolerance Group
www.gluten.net

National Foundation for Celiac Awareness
www.celiaccentral.org

Gluten-Free Prescription Drugs and Nutritional Supplements

Steve Plogsted, PharmD, runs a website (www.glutenfreedrugs.com) that serves as a good starting place to investigate the gluten content of prescription drugs.

With nutritional supplements, always check the label. Nutritional supplements are often labelled 'gluten-free', as well as listing the absence of other potential undesirable components, such as lactose.

Additional Recipes

Cookbooks in the low-carbohydrate and 'paleo' diets overlap to a great extent with the sorts of foods advocated in this cookbook. Their recipes are wheat-free and focus on real food ingredients.

Just be careful: some of the recipes in these cookbooks tend to use unhealthy sweeteners such as maple syrup, honey and agave, or occasionally rely too heavily on 'safe' starches like sweet potatoes or yams and rice. These carbohydrate sources are indeed safer than wheat and sugar, but they are not entirely healthy when consumed in larger quantities than a 120ml (4fl oz) serving.

Likewise, be careful with gluten-free cookbooks, as they often use unhealthy gluten-free replacements, such as rice flour, cornflour, potato flour, tapioca flour or premixed gluten-free flours. My advice: never use these flours. Avoid the recipes that call for them, and select only the ones that do not use these gluten-free flours.

Websites

Stay-at-home mum turned wheat/gluten-free, low-carb recipe writer Carolyn Ketchum provides great recipes accompanied by excellent photography.
www.alldayidreamaboutfood.com

Elana Amsterdam's beautiful and creative mostly almond flour–based recipes are featured on her website/blog, as well as in her cookbook listed in the next section.
www.elanaspantry.com

Formally trained in culinary arts, blogger Michelle provides great recipes that are free of wheat/gluten and corn.
www.glutenfreefix.com

Nutritionist Maria Emmerich is a wheat-free, limited-carbohydrate champion! She is among the few nutritionists who truly understand these important health concepts. The photography on her website is also stunningly beautiful. Maria's excellent cookbook is listed below.
www.mariahealth.blogspot.com

Books

The Art of Healthy Eating: Kids and *The Art of Healthy Eating: Sweets* by Maria Emmerich (CreateSpace, 2011)

Eat Like a Dinosaur: Recipe and Guidebook for Gluten-Free Kids by The Paleo Parents (Victory Belt Publishing, 2012)

Everyday Paleo by Sarah Fragoso (Victory Belt Publishing, 2011)

500 Paleo Recipes by Dana Carpender (Fair Winds Press, 2012)

The G-Free Diet: A Gluten-Free Survival Guide by Elisabeth Hasselbeck (Center Street, 2011)

Gather: The Art of Paleo Entertaining by Hayley Mason and Bill Staley (Victory Belt Publishing, 2013)

The Gluten-Free Almond Flour Cookbook by Elana Amsterdam (Celestial Arts, 2009)

The Gluten-Free Asian Kitchen by Laura B. Russell (Celestial Arts, 2011)

The Gluten-Free Bible: The Thoroughly Indispensable Guide to Negotiating Life without Wheat by Jax Peters Lowell (Holt Paperbacks, 2005)

The Gluten-Free Edge: Get Skinny the Gluten-Free Way! by Gini Warner and Chef Ross Harris (Adams Media, 2011)

Grain-Free Gourmet by Jodi Bager and Jenny Lass (Whitecap Books Ltd., 2010)

The Healthy Gluten-Free Life by Tammy Credicott (Victory Belt Publishing, 2012)

Make It Paleo by Bill Staley and Hayley Mason (Victory Belt Publishing, 2011)

Nutritious and Delicious by Maria Emmerich (Self, 2012)

1001 Low-Carb Recipes by Dana Carpender (Fair Winds Press, 2010)

Paleo Comfort Foods by Julie and Charles Mayfield (Victory Belt Publishing, 2011)

Paleo Cooking from Elana's Pantry by Elana Amsterdam (Ten Speed Press, 2013)

The Paleo Diet and *The Paleo Diet Cookbook* by Loren Cordain (Houghton Mifflin Harcourt 2010)

Practical Paleo by Diane Sanfilippo (Victory Belt Publishing, 2012)

The Primal Blueprint Cookbook by Mark Sisson and Jennifer Meier (Primal Nutrition, 2010)

More *Wheat Belly* Resources

Wheat Belly (Rodale, 2011)

This is the original book, released in August 2011, that details all the reasons why humans have no business eating modern wheat.

The Wheat Belly Blog, Facebook page and YouTube videos provide ongoing discussions about many issues relevant to wheat and living wheat free, as well as real stories of people who have discovered this lifestyle. I also post new recipes here.

Many articles, podcasts and TV interviews are archived on the blog.
www.wheatbellyblog.com
www.facebook.com/pages/Wheat-Belly
www.youtube.com/user/wheatbelly

Wheat-Free Research and Education Foundation

This is the organization I've helped establish that will, in the future, fund research, provide education, and help inform the public about the need to recognize the dangers of wheat consumption and the health benefits of ridding your life of it.
www.wheatfreeref.org

INDEX

Underscored page references indicate boxed text. An asterisk(*) indicates that photographs appear in the colour insert pages.